Your Weight is not the Problem

For anyone who has struggled with their weight due to a toxic, yo-yo relationship with diets.

It's time to break up with that loser.

Your Weight is not the Problem

A simple, no-diet plan for healthy habits that stick

Lyndi Cohen

murdoch books

Sydney | London

Published in 2023 by Murdoch Books, an imprint of Allen & Unwin

Murdoch Books Australia
Cammeraygal Country
83 Alexander Street, Crows Nest NSW 2065
Phone: +61 (0)2 8425 0100
murdochbooks.com.au
info@murdochbooks.com.au

Murdoch Books UK
Ormond House, 26–27 Boswell Street, London WC1N 3JZ
Phone: +44 (0) 20 8785 5995
murdochbooks.co.uk
info@murdochbooks.co.uk

 A catalogue record for this book is available from the National Library of Australia

A catalogue record for this book is available from the British Library

ISBN 978 1 92261 649 4

Cover and text design by George Saad
Back cover photograph by Luca Prodigo

Typeset by Midland Typesetters
Printed and bound by CPI Group (UK) Ltd, Croydon, CR04YY

DISCLAIMER: The content presented in this book is meant for inspiration and informational purposes only. The author and publisher claim no responsibility to any person or entity for any liability, loss, or damage caused or alleged to be caused directly or indirectly as a result of the use, application, or interpretation of the material in this book.

Every reasonable effort has been made to trace the owners of copyright materials in this book, but in some instances this has proven impossible. The author(s) and publisher will be glad to receive information leading to more complete acknowledgements in subsequent printings of the book and in the meantime extend their apologies for any omissions.

We acknowledge that we meet and work on the traditional lands of the Cammeraygal people of the Eora Nation and pay our respects to their elders past, present and future.

10 9 8 7 6 5 4 3 2

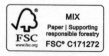

Contents

Introduction

On the diet treadmill

Chances are, you've tried countless diets. No one can say you haven't tried! In fact, you've been remarkably dedicated to weight loss. Take one look at your dieting resumè and, well, it's really quite impressive.

You've willingly signed up to grimy gyms without any windows and with way too many mirrors. You've batch cooked strange-smelling watery soups and drunk shakes in place of actual meals. You've beaten yourself up for eating too much and committed to starting from scratch many times over. At times, you've even felt guilty for eating a whole banana or an entire sandwich for fear of carbs (and then there were the fat- and sugar-phobic years)! You've counted points, calories or macros, diligently recording everything in a diary or app. And you've also pretended it was the dog who made those outrageously sour farts when, in fact, the smell came from your bum after eating too much of that weird protein powder stuff.

I know, I know. All those bloomin' mirrors are supposed to help with correct form, but who really wants to see themselves from 417 angles while flapping around like a drunken pigeon? Not me.

It was all very unfun. But you did it. You see, you really have been committed to this whole weight-loss thing. You deserve a frequent flyer discount card based on how much money you've handed over to diet companies and influential 'health gurus'. Even if you're new to this whole hating-your-body business, you've already spent far too many hours worrying about your weight or whether you're exercising enough. After all, it's immensely tricky to have a healthy relationship with your weight and food in a disordered society that thinks the most impressive thing a woman can be is thin.

And so, here you are. An incredibly smart, talented (at times mischievous) but always lovable human, who is able to accomplish anything you put your excellent noggin to. Except this. Your weight. It feels like the only thing you can't 'fix' or solve. And you wish you could, because you can't shake the feeling that your life would be better – and you would be happier – if your weight wasn't 'a problem'. The real issue is that you're stuck in the murky, contaminated waters of diet burnout. Each diet attempt has been less effective. Your motivation and willpower seem to whittle with each sad salad and globby chia seed you consume. You've never made it to the promised land of being thin-yet-somehow-curvy-in-just-right-places, and are you really willing to trudge through the dessertless dieting desert for another 40 years seeking it?

When your weight feels like a problem, you miss out on life. Dieting and 'trying to be good' keeps you stuck in the vicious ups and downs of yo-yo dieting. Ironically and frustratingly, you may be gaining weight with each failed attempt.[1] My dear client Natalia, who deserves a black belt for all her dieting experience, explained the conundrum: 'I've been dieting my whole life and I am the biggest that I have ever been. I feel like it is holding me back from doing things that I love. You feel you can't reach your potential until you shed the kilos or pounds. But I just keep getting further away the more I try.' Honestly? That's how it always felt for me, too.

My story

I was just five years old when my turbulent relationship with my body started. I was in ballet class, in a pink leotard, staring into the mirror when I noticed it. Where the other girls had straight-up-and-down bodies, I had a little tummy and thighs that touched. It was the beginning of feeling like my body was flawed.

PSA: the BMI is bullshit. We'll talk about that later in the book.

By age 11, I truly believed my weight was a major problem, despite being in the healthy weight range for my BMI. I felt that I wasn't going to be good enough until I weighed less, and it seemed the rest of the world agreed with me. I was told 'you'd be so pretty if you lost weight' so many times that I started to believe it.

So my parents took me to a nutritionist. The nutritionist under-stood my request. I wanted to be thin – and she was willing to help me subscribe to this ideal. She put me on a meal plan, which she pinky-promised wasn't a diet (even though it certainly was) then promptly instructed me to weigh out my food. Ha! There was no conversation about body image, about what it actually means to be healthy, or warnings about how dieters are significantly more likely to develop an eating disorder or struggle with their weight as adults.[2]

On my first very prescriptive, restricted 'healthy eating approach', I went to bed at night with a calorie-counting book, calculating whether or not I'd been 'good' or 'bad' that day. In addition to the regular weigh-ins at the nutritionist's office, I became obsessed with weighing myself. When I lost weight, I was elated and very proud. Everyone told me I was a good girl! The praise for losing weight reinforced my belief that I wasn't good enough as I was and that changing my body would help me to be more likeable. Better. Prettier! Worthier. And oh, how I wanted that. When I gained weight or even simply didn't lose any, I was distraught. My social currency was losing weight and I felt bankrupt. My sense of self was based on whether I lost or gained weight and whether I disappointed my family, my nutritionist and myself.

And sure enough, with time, the diets I stuck to so conscientiously stopped being effective. I ate what I was supposed to but I stopped losing weight. 'I've been so good this week,' I told my group leader at our public weigh-in, after meticulously tracking points and sticking to 'free' foods all week to dull the intense hunger pangs. 'Well, you must have cheated,' she told me in front of the whole group. 'The scales don't lie.' I somehow managed not to burst into tears until after I got into the car, the shame hot inside me. I was 14 years old.

Soon after, I started binge eating. While I was willing to calorie-control (aka starve) my way to weigh less, my body had an inbuilt protective mechanism to keep me from self-sacrificing. My body feared there was a famine so, when it finally got access to food, I felt compelled to uncontrollably eat as much as I could before it 'ran out'.

I gained weight quickly. My family was alarmed and didn't know what to do with me. I felt like such a disappointment, ashamed for being out of control with food. I was told I looked puffy, like an overly inflated balloon. By now my relationship with food was completely screwed up. Unhealthy and disordered. But on the outside, my ballooning weight was seen to be the real problem. And heartbreakingly, the harder I tried to lose weight, the more I ended up secretly bingeing on bowls of cereal, loaves of bread or peanut butter by the spoonful (which was always followed by crushing guilt and girl-scout promises to do better tomorrow).

When it came to binge eating, my body didn't discriminate. I'd devour 'forbidden' foods like cookies-and-cream ice cream straight from the tub just as readily as I'd gorge on healthy foods like cucumbers, berries or yoghurt. My body craved the things I was depriving it of. Calories. Food. Energy! The more intense my emotional eating episode or my binge was, the harder I'd double down on my dieting efforts in an attempt to regain control. This left me stuck in the vicious cycle of yo-yo dieting, eating well during the week then binge eating on the weekends only to have to start a new diet every Monday.

I wouldn't go to social events where I'd be forced to watch all my friends eat foods I wasn't allowed to eat, while I was ordering vegetables and dip (the dish I'd decided was the lowest in calories). I'd lie in bed at night doing mental arithmetic to assess what I'd eaten that day, and wondering how I could be 'better' tomorrow. I was so desperate to please that I once cut my hair in order to try to weigh less at a check-in appointment with my nutritionist.

But because I wasn't thin, no one thought I had a relationship-with-food problem. The more weight I gained, the more my dieting was encouraged, which only put my weight goals further out of reach. And my disordered eating thrived. Until the age of 21 this continued: being controlled by food, guilt and shame. All the while, my weight increased while the real problem was never treated.

The never-ending dieting rollercoaster had me in a chokehold, and the crushing pressure to do it all left me completely overwhelmed. I knew what I 'should' be eating, but why couldn't I stick to it? It turns out there wasn't anything wrong with my self-control. And there's nothing wrong with yours either.

Health has become too hard

Health has become synonymous with perfect eating. We think of being healthy and imagine supplements, organic food, 5 am wake-ups, crop tops, flat stomachs and impressive bowls filled with perfectly nourishing macro-balanced foods. Or we picture a perfect calorie-controlled diet where we stick to diet rules like 'don't eat too many carbs' and carefully count how many grams of protein we have left. Any deviation from this plan makes us feel like we've messed up.

If we eat a chocolate biscuit or an innocent piece of bread, we think we've 'ruined it' for the day. May as well finish the packet to start fresh again tomorrow, right? Not only is dieting expensive but for most of us it's utterly unsustainable. Why? Because it's making us *un*healthy.

We think our weight is the problem and dieting is the solution. But in reality, the more we focus on trying to lose weight, the harder it is to instill sustainable and healthy habits that really help our bodies feel good. Anyone who has ever dieted will know how frustrating, stressful and life-impacting this situation is.

Also, I know I'm not the only one who is completely burnt out simply by trying to do it all. Now that I'm a mum, there is even less time in the day – once you take into account the mental load of trying to work out what's for dinner every freakin' night, keep the house clean, exercise regularly, drink eight glasses of water, respond to emails, have a social life, be a good friend, sister, partner and daughter, all while not having a mental breakdown. It's tiring. It feels like my needs are constantly on the backburner and I'm burning the candle at both ends to serve others. There's far too much scrolling, comparing, being busy and saying yes when I really need to say no.

All this people-pleasing and striving leaves us feeling depleted and, quite frankly, annihilated by the relentlessness of it all. And that's before the pressure to fit into the same size clothes you wore in high school or before you had kids. It's a lot.

I'm the first to admit that I prioritise finding my child's stuffed whale amid the pyramid pile of dirty laundry before caring for my body, wellbeing, interests and mental health. Sometimes, I get to the end of the day before I realise I've been holding in a poo for hours! Was I waiting for someone to give me permission to go to the toilet? My husband doesn't suffer like this: he happily takes a luxurious 45 minutes to sit on the loo without a tiny human watching. Bliss! Why do we spend so much time ensuring the ones we love are well fed and cared for, or saying yes to plans we don't really want to follow through with, and constantly allow ourselves to come last? And it sure doesn't help that 'self-care' is pushed at us when what we really need is community care. It's no wonder we are Generation Burnout.

Perhaps you're like me. Someone who kills every orchid I've ever owned. But also, someone who is a failed perfectionist. Perfectionism tells us that if we can't do something perfectly, then it's not worth doing at all. But 'perfect eating' is the enemy of healthy eating. The result is being all-or-nothing when it comes to health and constantly wishing we weighed less, but seemingly paralysed by overwhelm and diet burnout. There is another way.

If anyone can help me with the orchid-murdering situation, I'd be most grateful.

I reckon it's time to adopt a new way of thinking about food. And a kinder, better approach to health where we don't need to feel exhausted for simply existing. Don't you?

If dieting worked, wouldn't you be at your goal weight by now?

My ~~breaking point~~ life-saving moment

I was 21, in a change room at a clothing store, trying on an outfit for a friend's birthday party. Seeing myself in the mirror, a lump of deep loathing filled my throat. I felt disgusting. I hated myself so much I jumped in my car and drove straight to the doctor, completely distraught. Explaining my unhinged relationship with food and my body, I was immediately prescribed anti-anxiety medication and a new diet. While my attitude towards food had become unhealthy and very disordered, I was told that the scales meant I didn't have an eating disorder. In other words, I was too heavy to consider that. My weight, not how and why I was eating, was the problem. And dieting was supposedly the solution.

Rather than recognising that I was struggling with disordered eating, the doctor suggested I try another diet that his wife was currently having some success with. Oh geez. I couldn't escape diet culture even inside my doctor's office. Weight stigma meant my concerns around eating were dismissed and instead of receiving the treatment I needed, I was told to just . . . try harder.

'But I have tried!' I wanted to yell. I really had tried so damn hard, for so many years and it just hadn't worked. Not only that, but I was now buying the biggest clothes I'd ever purchased even after a decade of dedication to dieting. I'd sacrificed my mental health and my social life, and developed an eating disorder in pursuit of my goal weight. Yet, it still wasn't enough.

This was my ~~breaking point~~ life-saving light bulb moment. Because it was the final push I needed to realise that this approach of 'trying to be good' and 'more willpower' and 'just eat less' wasn't working. Even after total commitment to it.

Finally, it dawned on me that I was never going to look like the women plastered up (for fitspo) on my vision board. I was never going to have a 'perfect' body. Maybe it was time to aim to be healthy instead. I wanted to feel comfortable in my clothes and normal around food. With this realisation, there was huge relief to know that I didn't have to keep striving to weigh less all the time.

Healing my relationship with food

By this point, I was an accredited practising dietitian and nutritionist, freshly graduated from university with my Bachelor of Nutrition and Dietetics. I'm the first to admit that I'd chosen this profession for all the wrong reasons. When I started studying, I'd rationalised that being a nutritionist would be the perfect job to help me stay thin. Being the right weight was part of the job description, wasn't it? And it would force me to diet forever.

But want to know the interesting thing? By studying nutrition, I learned that food is so much more than the calories you consume or what you weigh. Woah. And health can be measured in so many other ways beyond waist circumference or BMI – mindblowing stuff. Once I graduated, I found myself in a personal crisis. I knew I had to work on my own relationship with food before I could start helping others.

Following that disastrous visit to my doctor I decided to shift my focus away from my lifelong efforts to weigh less. I threw my scales out: an exceptionally liberating moment! Instead of using weight as the metric for my success, I focused my mental energy on how my body *felt* rather than how it looked. Instead of shunning 'bad' foods, I chose foods I wanted to eat more of, to crowd onto my plate. Instead of following rigid diet rules, I collected new healthy habits I could actually stick to. This book details the steps I took – and that you can take, too – to stop dieting and form a trusting, healthy relationship with food.

Fear not, I did change doctors after this, finding a professional who cared more about my health than my BMI.

The surprising result of the whole hitting-rock-bottom-then-quitting-diets thing is that I ended up losing 20 kilograms (44 lb) over four years. But this only happened when I stopped frantically trying to change my weight. The very thing I had chased all those years was the unexpected outcome of letting go of the perfectionism and obsession with my weight. It was simply a by-product of focusing on my health and my relationship with food.

Healing your relationship with food

Your weight isn't the problem you've been told it is. And fixating on it is making it harder to eat healthily, to move your body with enjoyment and to like what you see in the mirror. As my wonderful client Kate told me, 'I have always thought I've had a problem with my weight, for as long as I can remember – 30-plus years. But a problem with my RELATIONSHIP with food? That is new. This feels different!'

This book will help you shift your focus away from your weight – from the negative thinking that is sabotaging your health – and adopt a new approach to wellness that is a lot more achievable.

To be clear, this isn't a weight-loss book, though you may end up losing weight as a result of the things you learn as you read this book. Then again, you might not. The goal is to help you adopt healthy habits, without the dieting noise, allowing your weight to find its own sweet spot. Those who are underweight may even gain weight.

I don't know about you, but I've wasted too much time, money and energy buying diet books and programs that have failed me. I don't want this to be another failed thing for you to add to your already extensive list.

We'll begin in Part 1 by dismantling diet thinking. We'll uncover the psychology behind weight loss and the annoying physiological changes that make it damn impossible for you and 95 per cent of us to successfully lose weight and keep it off with diets.[3] I want you to feel excellent in your body and have the energy to do the things you love. This book is more than just diet-bashing and calling out wellness wankery.

Though there's a bit of that in here for sure!

This isn't a quick fix either. If, like me, you've been dieting for years (or maybe even decades like many of my clients), it's going to take more than a 12-week challenge to rejig your thinking and transform your life. Instead, we'll dive into the real reasons why you feel like you can't stop snacking or feel addicted to sugar. I'll pass on the learning I've gained from over a decade working as a dietitian, helping patients and clients find real health and regain freedom around their weight and food. I'll give you a new, more sustainable approach to food, weight and your body. You simply have to take what works for you and chuck out what doesn't.

Hint: It's probably different from what you've been taught elsewhere.

Together, we'll relearn the basics of being healthy while flipping our middle fingers to perfectionism, that pesky monster that makes healthy eating so much trickier than it needs to be. Plus, I'll share some hard-earned wisdom that I know will help you add micro-habits so that you can build a healthier life. I'll spare you the too-hard, who-the-heck-can-even-do-that suggestions. (I'm the first to roll my eyes at those 'hacks'.)

Plus, there'll be no woowoo or things that can't be substantiated with clinical evidence or research. As a healthcare professional, I feel a responsibility to use science to chip away at nutrition nonsense, one bullsh*t brick at a time. You bet I'll be sharing important tools to help you deal with common pitfalls, such as perfectionism, comparison and body hatred.

The end result? Feeling more comfortable in your body. Healthy eating that comes more easily. Exercising because you enjoy it, not as punishment for eating. More consistency! No more starting from scratch every Monday, falling off the bandwagon or feeling like your weight is a lifelong struggle. Plus, you'll gain freedom from self-blame and learn how to forgive yourself for not being perfect. You'll get a whole lot more headspace once your thoughts aren't plagued by how much you hate your body or regret what you ate yesterday. Oh, how very lovely! And how very well deserved.

> Consistency – the most crucial (yet often elusive) ingredient in healthy living.

You can be healthy without sacrificing 95 per cent of your life to weigh five per cent less.

This book will also explore why we feel tired all the freakin' time and oh, so burned out. It takes a look into what happens when you prioritise what other people think about your body over how you feel inside it, and when you spend more time taking care of others than yourself. The result is fatigue; feeling like we're endlessly chasing an unreachable goal and can never be good enough.

This may be one of the reasons we frequently feel overwhelmed and struggle with consistency (along with the constant social-media doomscrolling, an energy exchange that we'll also chat about later). And so, this book will offer some new stuff to guide you as you learn to prioritise yourself and rebuild your energy reserves, the ultimate currency you trade in. This means more energy, and less lying in bed at night feeling guilty for eating (or existing as an imperfect human). You'll feel more comfortable in your body, gain freedom from food and be able to focus on health without obsession. Think: you will be exercising because you enjoy it, eating healthily without stressing and embracing your perfectly imperfect body.

The truth is you can't live a full life on an empty stomach, my friend. Or be the enigmatic, sensational human you're meant to be when every thought comes back to worrying about your weight.

Introduction

No one will stand up at your funeral and talk about your stomach pouch or whether or not you had cellulite or scrawny arms (and if they do, your friends are shit). It's time to embrace a new approach to health where you stop thinking of your weight as the problem, freeing you up to adopt all the delicious, sticky, healthy habits that will actually help you feel good (no, amazing!) in your body.

It doesn't matter how many years you've been dieting for. It's never too late to build a healthier relationship with food. And I want to help you do that.

Big love,

Lyndi

Before we begin

In this impressive masterpiece of a book (my mum's words, not mine), you'll read stories from real, actual, living, human people. You'll read anecdotes shared by my clients that I've gathered over my career, from my private practice days and now via my online program Keep It Real. Plus, you'll read case studies and interesting tidbits I've safely stored while doing this whole 'being a dietitian who genuinely likes people and helps them avoid the diet trap' thing. While I've changed the names of my clients for anonymity, I've done minimal editing to their words. That felt important. You see, I desperately want you to know that these problems are universal, felt by many, and in no way are they a reflection of your worth, character or willpower. You're wonderful. Anyone who matters would agree.

Alrighty then. Enough small talk. Time to crack this puppy open.

Part 1:
Free Yourself From Diets

Building a solid foundation for your new relationship with food and your body (something you so deserve) is very important. You've got to tell diet nonsense to get stuffed and demolish your old way of thinking. In Part 1, we'll be clearing out diet clutter to spark a whole lot more joy as well as detoxing the wellness wankery from your lovely headspace. (It's the only detox I'll ever recommend.) We'll be laying the foundations for your hierarchy of healthy habits (see Chapter 4) that will establish the structure you need. The goal? To build a healthier approach to food and your body on a rock-solid foundation.

Chapter 1.

You haven't failed at diets. Diets have failed you.

You might already know that diets suck.
You've done enough of them to realise this! Like your
ex from high-school days, they're flaky, ask for more
than they give and just aren't a viable long-term option.
And yet, many whip-smart, wonderful people are
still dieting. So our first step is to take a look at what
diets do to our bodies and clear out some persistent
nutrition nonsense.

How diets fail you

Weight-loss researchers have been sounding the alarm bell for quite some time about the fact that diets are failing us. Scientists conducted a high-quality meta-analysis (a systematic review of randomised control trials) in 2014.[1] After reviewing all the evidence, the team concluded with brutal honesty that current weight-loss methods Just. Aren't. Working. They pleaded for better strategies. From what they could see, the current diet methods being pushed only lead to minuscule reductions in weight loss, along with a side serving of weight regain and weight cycling. The smart people conducting these studies were practically shouting into a megaphone, saying, 'Better approaches are needed!' And yet, the same old shamey diet advice keeps being dished out: 'Eat less. Move more. Count calories. Try harder!'

Weight cycling is when you lose weight, regain it, lose weight again and keep doing this forever and ever.

Another study published in the *American Journal of Public Health* followed thousands of people (76,704 men and 99,791 women) over ten years.[2] It showed that the chance of someone in a larger body successfully losing weight and keeping it off with diet and exercise was really, really, outrageously low. The study found that the probability of losing weight and keeping it off with diet for an obese person was one in 210 for men and one in 124 for women. When someone is morbidly obese, it becomes five to ten times less likely! It's often quoted that 95 per cent of diets fail in the long term,[3] but this research pegs that number at closer to 99 per cent.

Regardless of our weight, we're all doing the diet thing and hating our bodies anyway. When I asked my Instagram followers if they thought they'd be happier if they weighed less, more than 3500 people responded and 82 per cent said yes. Eighty per cent said their weight feels like a constant struggle. According to another survey, 39 per cent

You haven't failed at diets. Diets have failed you.

23

of women said concerns about their weight or what they eat interferes with their happiness.[4] That's sad. But also relatable, perhaps?

My client Barbara, 61, says she's been fighting against her body for as long as she can remember. 'It's been a lifetime of dieting for me, followed by going back to old ways and night-time bingeing. Success for weeks followed by failure weeks later. Weight going down feels great, only to go up again. Often my mood will depend on my weight! If I feel and look thin, I feel good, happy and confident. When my weight is up, I feel awful, angry with myself, tight in my clothes, etc. And the cycle goes on and on and on. I'm 61 years young and still fighting the weight fight.' If you aren't actively deciding to move away from dieting, you could spend the rest of your life stuck on the diet rollercoaster.

There are myriad ways diets kick you in the tits and rob you of hard-earned dimes and precious time. Here are just some of the ways diets epically fail you.

Diets lead to weight gain

It's not just that diets don't lead to weight loss. Statistically, dieting and diet rules lead to weight gain:[5] the very thing dieters fear the most! How sinister and unfair. Oh, the trickery. And yet, what a very typical 'diet' thing to do.

Why does this happen? There are many reasons. Typically, your body doesn't love being in a calorie deficit, so it may adapt. When your body fears that less energy is being provided than it needs to meet the requirements of day-to-day living, it can take action. Your body may start to slow your metabolism and increase your hunger (your body has a bag of tricks to help make this happen) to ensure it prevents further weight loss and promotes weight gain. Your body feels safer this way. This is often referred to as starvation mode, though I like to call it the 'survival switch'.[6] Later in the book, we'll talk about how to work with it, instead of against it. And it may be one of the reasons that explain why people regain weight after going on a diet.

In reality, many people gain even more weight after going on diets than they originally lost. In one study, researchers caught up with dieters three years after

It's tempting to hate starvation mode but it's probably the reason you're here today, as it's helped keep generations of humans alive during periods of food shortages. Believe it or not, it's a protective system.

they'd completed a weight-loss program to see how they were going.[7] It turns out only 12 per cent of the dieters had kept off at least three-quarters of the weight they had originally lost. Meanwhile, 40 per cent had gained back more weight than they lost during the diet. Hmmm. Another study looked at a smaller group of women and found that six months after finishing a diet they weighed on average 3.6 kilograms (8 lb) more than before they dieted.[8] Further work by researchers investigating diabetes suggests that only 19 per cent of people will be able to maintain at least ten per cent of their weight loss after five years.[9]

Weight gain after dieting is a common pattern (and is probably underestimated because long-term follow up of weight-loss programs is pathetically low).[10]

Rachel is a mum of two girls who experienced this post-diet weight regain first hand. 'I started dieting when I was maybe 15 years old. I have had a strange relationship with food since. It has become increasingly worse over the past two years as I tried to lose the last five kilograms [11 lb] of weight from having my second child. I have tried intermittent fasting, no carbs, low carbs, healthy fats . . . only to actually gain another eight kilograms [18 lb]. I now have no idea what I should eat, so sometimes I just don't bother cooking for myself. I want to feel that I can go to the beach next summer and not feel awful. I want to be in family photos, rather than be the one who takes them to avoid looking at myself.' Not only is Rachel now confused about what she 'should' eat, she's also too paralysed by indecision to do anything about it and she's gained more weight as a result of dieting than if she had simply done nothing.

This is a common tale. Dieting in your teens makes you more likely to be categorised as overweight or obese as an adult,[11] and women who start dieting before age 14 tend to have higher BMIs.[12] While teens who are overweight are more likely to go on a diet, many start dieting when they are considered in the 'normal' BMI weight range. And teens who diet are twice as likely to be overweight as adults compared with teens who didn't diet, regardless of starting weight.[13]

On the flipside, a ten-year study showed that folks who have never dieted (and have regular eating habits) are more likely to maintain their weight. And the more diets you go on? The greater your chances

You haven't failed at diets. Diets have failed you.

25

of being obese.[14] Oh, and not only does dieting lead to weight gain, but it also makes you more likely to have disordered eating.[15]

In the long term, dieting is more likely to lead to weight gain than weight loss. A review published in 2013 found that recent dieting seemed to be a predictor for weight gain.[16] That's the reward you get for all that effort you put in! You get an A+ for dedication and a lifetime of trying to 'fix' your weight problem. And yet, for some reason, two-thirds of people still believe dieting is an effective way to lose weight.[17] It's not. It's really, truly, scientifically not. Do you think you can start to accept that?

Dieting is more likely to lead to weight gain than weight loss.

Diets increase cravings

In an annoying twist, dieting increases our cravings for the very things we're trying to avoid.[18] Those forbidden foods become tastier, more interesting and exciting. It's true that some diets can lead to a decrease in cravings,[19] but that's only while you're sticking to the rules. Given the unsustainability of diets, when you inevitably do stop following them, you're left with increased cravings compared with before you started the diet. This is just one of the mechanisms of how diets lead to weight regain and, often, out-of-control eating.

We want what we can't have, right? To test this theory, let's do a little experiment: for the next minute, put this book down and, whatever you do, don't think about feet. Don't picture feet. Don't imagine them. Keep the image of a foot or feet out of your mind. Alright, time to do the experiment! One minute. Let's go.

How did you go? If you're like most people, you probably found it almost impossible not to think about feet during the test. Why? It seems our humble yet brilliant human brains have a hard time not locking on to the thing being fixated on, even if it's mentioned in the negative. Don't look down. Don't think about your ex.

Social psychologist Daniel Wegner was pretty fascinated by this idea. Do we really have control over what we think about? Maybe not, according to his infamous 'white bear' study, first published in 1987.[20] He asked participants to talk in a stream of consciousness for five minutes, with only one rule: don't think about a white bear! And if they did think about a white bear, he asked them to ring a bell.

The participants rang the bell an average of once per minute, showing just how tough it is to not think about something you've been told not to think about.

The hypothesis behind why this happens? While one part of your brain is trying its best not to think about a white bear or feet, the other part of your brain is constantly checking in to make sure you haven't yet thought of either of those things.

This – along with such feelings of restriction as 'everyone else is allowed to eat yummy food but I'm not' – may explain what happens in your brain when you try to avoid a bunch of foods you've been told are

How diet companies work

Dieting for your weight is like putting concealer on a zit. It's going to cover up the thing you're self-conscious about, but it's going to make the situation a whole lot worse in the long term. Like a red pimple emerging angrier after it's infected, your relationship with food will likely take a pounding with each diet attempt you chase after.

Diet companies don't want you to know that diets don't work. They need you to rebound! The success of a diet company relies on you returning again as a customer. If they fixed the actual problem, you wouldn't continue to pay them money. You wouldn't be back counting points for the fifth time, or buying yet another book on intermittent fasting. They would have a business model but they wouldn't be the billion-dollar enterprises that many of them are. As of 2021, the American diet industry was estimated to be worth $72.6 billion.[21]

Exactly how much does it cost to lose weight by buying into the promises of diet companies? To lose five kilograms (11 lb) with WeightWatchers will cost you around $755. And if you're using a drug such as orlistat, it could cost $2730.[22] We know that most of us will lose and regain the same weight many time over in our lifetimes, likely spending tens of thousands of dollars on impermanent results. As a result, we end up fuelling diet companies with more money, which feeds the industry to sell us even more compelling advertising.

catastrophic for your wellbeing. Don't eat ice cream. Don't think about bread. No pasta for you! Chocolate is a no-go!! Don't think about all the things you're missing out on!!! It's a wonder that we don't end up face-planting into the pantry more often.

If avoiding foods makes you crave them more, how do you eat healthily without creating a list of forbidden foods? Can you eat well without applying a gajillion diet rules? You can, with healthy habits done right. We'll tackle how to adopt this divine hierarchy in Part 2.

Diets lead to food obsession

Then there's the overwhelming obsession with food that comes from being on a diet. The landmark Minnesota Starvation Experiment is a perfect example.[23] In the study, 36 male volunteers were placed on a semi-starvation diet (not dissimilar to a modern weight-loss diet). The results were fascinating and quite pivotal. Once placed on a restricted diet (1,570 calories a day, which was about half the recommended intake for the male volunteers; the equivalent dietary restriction for a female would be a 1200 calorie diet, something many dieters would be familiar with), the men noticed a decrease in sex drive, strength and stamina. They also reported fatigue, irritability, apathy and depression. Relatable for any dieter, isn't it? It's hard to be your best self when your brain and body are starved of energy.

This is an outrageously unethical experiment by today's standards, but somehow it passed the test in 1944 (during World War II).

But what was incredibly profound was how these men now found themselves completely preoccupied with food. Totally and utterly obsessed! Before the study, food was just food – something yummy that provided fuel – but when semi-starved? It consumed their thoughts and even their dreams. They would fantasise about food, imagining what they'd eat if they could. They wanted to read books about food, look at food photos and talk about food with the other research participants.

Perhaps this has happened to you, too, when you've been on a diet? You notice your thoughts keep coming back to food all day. You see, dieting makes food you were previously indifferent to become quite 'interesting'.

This phenomenon may explain why a friend or colleague who is on a diet feels compelled to brag and tell everyone about their weight-loss pursuit. While we may feel a twinge of jealousy when they talk about how much weight they've lost, what if we started to see this constant diet chatter for what it might be: a clue that they may be starving their body and have become obsessed with food as a result. Your friend boasting about their weight loss isn't inspirational. It could be a symptom of dieting and disorder.

Dieting makes food more desirable

The other quirky thing that happens to your brain on a diet is that not only are you now obsessed by certain foods (or all food, in general) but when you do eventually eat, the food is now more appealing than it was before you went on a diet.

Do you like macaroni and cheese? I sure do. Some smart researchers did a delightfully interesting study using this delicious comfort food.[24] They gave participants an unlimited supply of macaroni and cheese to eat every day for the length of the study and measured how much they ate. In the beginning of the study, they found the participants ate quite a bit. With newfound freedom, they were excited by the chance to eat this delicious food! The bowl of cheesy macaroni was highly 'interesting' for them.

But as the study carried on, the participants became less and less excited by the idea of eating macaroni and cheese. As you can imagine, it became less enticing or exciting. That's because macaroni and cheese was allowed and highly available. It simply became yet another food they could eat. Now that this once-very-appealing food was something they knew they could eat whenever they wanted, it lost status. And appeal. The results showed that they ate far less macaroni and cheese as the study went on.

While this study might be taking it to the extreme, it's illustrating an important point. When you know that you can eat something you love whenever you like, it can reduce how enticing and 'interesting' it feels for you. Dieting does the opposite to your brain. It boosts obsession for food, especially the foods you love but you're meant to avoid. This might help explain why you have intense cravings for certain foods like chocolate, or why you overeat all foods, not just the forbidden ones. In Part 3 of this book, I'll go into more detail about how to shift away from restriction and food obsession so you can do the healthy stuff, without getting bogged down in nutrition noise.

Some signs you might be obsessed with food

* Once you start eating, you find it hard to stop.
* You lie in bed analysing what you ate that day.
* You map out – mentally, in an app or on paper – what you plan to eat in the future.
* You check the menu before you eat out to make sure there's something you will be able to eat.
* You feel guilty after eating.
* You love seeing a breakdown of others' 'day on a plate'.
* You see food ads on TV and wish you could eat the food.
* You plan out what you're going to eat at each meal.
* You feel jealous or envious when you see others eating.
* You record what you eat in a food diary.
* You love looking through recipes that you don't intend to cook.
* You enjoy watching other people eat.
* You love talking about or trading diet tips with friends or family.
* You don't understand how someone could 'forget' to eat.
* You feel the need to finish everything on your plate.

Failing diets crush your self worth

There's another dark side of diets. You start a new diet propelled by the belief that there is something wrong with your physical body, right? So when dieting doesn't work, you blame your internal self;[25] this is perhaps the most sinister of all the side effects. You believe you're weak. No self-control.

When a diet fails you, not only do you have your body to hate, but your self-worth, the very nature and essence of who you are as a person, is questioned. You begin to define yourself in black-and-white terms, dulling your already fragile sense of self-love. This is big stuff! It's not really just a simple, innocent thing.

When a diet fails you, not only do you have your body to hate, but your self-worth, the very nature and essence of who you are as a person, is questioned. In your mind, being thin is the basis of being accepted, loved and worthy enough.

People who have never had a 'weight problem', or haven't felt that there was something wrong with their body, might struggle to understand how big a deal this is for many of us. During my dieting years, insulting my weight was the one thing that would reliably bring me to tears. Worrying about your weight isn't frivolous. We joke about it – 'Diet starts Monday!' – but it's serious stuff. In our minds, being thin is the basis of being accepted, loved and worthy enough. This is why we chase our dream body with fervour even after countless previous failed attempts. It's not just vanity, though probably there is a peppering of that if we're honest! What we're really seeking is acceptance.

I'm not a teary person (unless I watch *Marley & Me* or *The Notebook*, in which case I'm a puddle).

A client, Margot, 33, had a gastric sleeve applied, around the time of her 31st birthday. Before her weight loss, she had dated crappy, unreliable men who cancelled on her at the last minute, ghosted her and couldn't commit to a long-term relationship. She explained how because of her weight and the way that impacted her self-esteem, she had allowed men to treat her this way, continuing to tolerate shonky behaviour because she felt it was all she really deserved. It was only post-surgery that she realised – almost overnight – that she was no longer willing to accept being mistreated.

But here's the thing. You don't need to wait until you've lost weight to finally decide you're worthy of respect. You can't keep chasing self-acceptance through weight loss. You can reach a point where you feel happy with yourself, worthy and good enough. But it's not going to be the result of some dramatic body transformation.

It's a decision you make – something we'll talk about in detail in this book. Because at the core of it, it doesn't matter if you have a flatter stomach or neat, toned arms. If you go to bed at night hating yourself, then it's still a loss.

Honest diet ad

Oh hey there! Like 95 per cent of people, you'll probably regain the weight you lose on this diet.[26] Thanks, because we make more money each time you fail and have to restart. Selling you an unsustainable meal plan is very profitable for us. Oh, and by the way, we sell thinness, not health, so your mental wellbeing isn't really our concern. That's why we use before-and-after photos of people who temporarily lost weight with us (we can't show you what they look like now because . . . well, that would be bad for business). On that note, can you please take photos of yourself so we can use YOUR photos for OUR marketing purposes? It'll help motivate you, but only temporarily because hating yourself isn't actually sustainable motivation. Make sure you look sad with bad lighting in the 'before' photo and then happy in the 'after' photo. OK, great. Thank you, come again when you've put the weight back on. We know you will . . . Muahahaha!

Scenarios where diets work

Here's what the world fails to recognise. Diets might work in the short term. But they would only work in the long term if you were:

* a robot without human desires or a social life;
* a celebrity with a personal assistant, private chef and a gaggle of staff to lighten your load as you traipse through life;
* locked in a room and fed through a small hole for eternity (not recommended by myself or Rapunzel).

So while many diets might possibly work in an alternative universe where we are free from our own physiology, they do not work – long term – in the real world. There will always be another long weekend, office party, date night, wedding, engagement, Bat Mitzvah, Diwali festivities, Easter egg hunt or Christmas lunch on the horizon. And of course there are emotional stressors – such as financial hardship, injury, debilitating illness, moving house or a new job – that mean quick fixes are bound to fail.

Many diets encourage you to starve yourself under the guise of health, convincing you that you can thrive on a 1200 calorie-a-day diet even though that's the bare minimum you need to survive and the recommended calorie intake for a toddler. Drinking shakes instead of eating food and pretending it's health? No, thank you.

Ultimately, diets fail to do what they say they will on the box: help you lose weight and keep it off. Instead, they set you up for yo-yo dieting by promising you transformations and selling you extreme, unmaintainable aspirations.

Are you accidentally dieting?

We all know what a diet is, right? They're generally easy to spot: conventional diets often include the word 'diet' in their name. Gotcha, you slippery beast! They will often give you a meal plan prescribing what to eat at every moment of the day, based on either calories, points or macros. You might be asked to record what you eat diligently in an app or paper diary to 'stay on track'. And of course, no diet is complete without a list of foods or nutrients to avoid. It could be sugar, gluten, carbs or fat. Basically the same diets get regurgitated every few years simply under a different name: think Atkins, Paleo, Keto. Same shit, different names: now for the new low price of just eleventy nine dollars! Alternatively the diet could be none of those things but tell you to starve yourself for whole chunks of time (confusing, I know). Intermittent fasting is simply self-inflicted starvation sold to us with some clever rebranding. These traditional diets are obvious. We know they are diets. But could you be on a diet without even realising it?

Here are some sneaky phrases you might utter if you're accidentally dieting:
* Oh no! I'm not dieting, I'm just trying to be good.
* I just eat everything in moderation.
* I'm just trying to eat clean.
* I'm only avoiding sugar for a little while.
* I have to watch what I eat.
* This is naughty food!
* I really shouldn't eat that.
* I've been so good this week.

All these socially acceptable phrases can be code for 'I'm on a diet'. The fact is, while diets have gone out of fashion like monocles, mullets and those extra-large shoulder pads from the eighties that resemble postnatal maxi-pads, many people are doing diets in disguise.

And let me be clear here, lovely one. You're not to blame. You're smart. But diets? Oh, they're crafty critters. They really don't want you to know that they are, in fact, diets. Diet companies spend lots of money camouflaging their real identity: 'We're not a diet, we're a "healthy lifestyle approach".' Nowadays, it's become outrageously hard to avoid diet noise. But given that diets have a very poor long-term success rate, it's important to make sure you're not getting lured into another. Because I can think of 38,049 better things to waste your money, time and energy on than yet another failed diet attempt. A jetski, perhaps? A trip to Greece sounds nice!

Given that old-school diets with their plans, tracking systems and before-and-after photos are so obvious, why are so many intelligent humans accidentally dieting? The answer: diet rules. Think of diet rules as the crappy souvenirs you get after being a committed dieter. But unlike a cheap, flimsy Eiffel Tower keyring that falls apart as soon as you unpack your suitcase, diet rules stick around for as long as you let them. They cloud your brain. They take up precious headspace. And they make choosing what to eat overwhelming and guilt-laden.

What are diet rules?

Diet rules are the residue left over from past diet attempts. Even after you've stopped attending meetings, weigh-ins and sticking to the meal plan, diet rules stick around like guests at a dinner party who can't take the hint to leave (even after you've put on your pyjamas and turned off the lights). They're also the by-product of reading and absorbing the diet advice that's often found in magazines, newspapers and social media. Sadly, taking on more of this diet advice makes you three times more likely to do unhealthy things to your body, such as taking laxatives, smoking or skipping meals, all in the name of 'health'.[27]

Like break-ups and underwear that insists on riding up your bum, diets (along with their unwanted lovechild 'diet rules') suck. You might be dieting without realising it if you eat according to portion size rather than your hunger level; if you weigh yourself daily, or multiple times a day; or if you often feel guilty when you eat 'bad' foods, or too many carbs, or food that isn't 'clean'. Most of us have plenty of niggling diet rules (sometimes hundreds) floating about in our brains. For chronic dieters who have done many diets over plenty of years or decades, there can be a real build-up of these pesky rules. Many of them end up contradicting each other as diet and superfood trends have evolved. Combine this with the constant nutrition noise in the media and it's no wonder food and eating healthily feels deeply confusing. And too hard.

So, what exactly is a diet rule? I'm glad you asked. Here are a bunch of diet rules I crowdsourced from my wonderful Instagram followers, who were asked to submit their most prevalent diet rules. This is (sadly) not an exhaustive list of diet rules, but it'll kick things off!

Common diet rules include:
* Fruit has too much sugar.
* Bread and pasta should be avoided.
* Don't have carbs after 5 pm.
* Don't eat bread or carbs more than once a day.
* A sandwich has too many carbs.
* Pasta is a treat.
* Brush your teeth so you don't feel like eating.
* If you're hungry, drink water because you might just be thirsty.
* Stick to portion sizes.
* You can't go back for seconds even if you're hungry.
* Women shouldn't eat as much as men.
* You're only allowed 100–150 calories per snack.
* You can only eat 12 nuts at a time.
* You can't eat protein and carbs in the same meal.
* You must eat protein and carbs in the same meal.
* Stick to 'low sugar' fruit like berries.
* Sauces contain lots of hidden sugar.
* Don't eat chemicals.
* Only eat foods you can pronounce.
* Gluten is bad for you.
* Coffee is bad for you.
* Coffee is good for you.

You haven't failed at diets. Diets have failed you.

Exhausting isn't it? Now imagine all of these contradicting diet rules ricocheting around your brain every time you try to make a food decision. Seemingly simple daily tasks like buying groceries, choosing from a menu, deciding what to cook for dinner or trying to determine whether you've eaten enough food suddenly become far more complicated. So much for the idea that diet rules 'help' you.

These rules take up space in your brain rent-free, without you knowing they're there, so the first step to creating a healthy relationship with food is to become aware of all the diet rules you subscribe to.

✎ Identify your diet rules

1. Pick up your phone (or a pen and paper if you're old school) and start a new note, titled 'Diet Rules'. Or 'Reasons I feel crazy around food' will work just fine as well.

2. Jot down any diet rules you can think of that you currently have, using the list above as a guide. Try to note down diet rules that you currently subscribe to along with the diet rules you believe would work if you 'could only stick to them'.

3. Over the next week (or a longer or shorter time, as you need), try to notice diet rules as they come up, during meals or when you're lying in bed. Add them to the list. This list is going to become an important piece of the puzzle, helping you free yourself from diets.

To download an easy-to-use (and printer-friendly) PDF with all the activities that you'll find in this book, head to *lyndicohen.com/bookresources*.

Diet rules aren't helping you

But surely these rules are helpful and healthy? Trying to eat the 'right' food and avoid the 'bad' ones is good for me? You might wonder, 'If I didn't do these things, I'd dive head-first into a bathtub of melted chocolate and may never come out!' Hold up. Before you imagine yourself as a human-sized Easter bunny, let's consider an alternative. What if these diet rules aren't helping you eat healthily and maintain your weight? Instead, they're the very thing leading to out-of-control eating, all-or-nothing thinking and your yo-yoing weight 'problem'.

If your diet rules worked, would you have reached your goal weight by now?

I really do get it. Diet rules help you feel like you've got control over food. So whenever you've shame-spiralled after eating more than you planned over a long weekend or at the holiday buffet, you've returned to these trusty diet rules to get 'back on track'. After all, when you do follow them, you feel better. Clients have told me that 'it works as long as I stick to it' or 'I lost so much weight when I did it, but I just can't get back into that mindset'. Here's the thing: if something only works temporarily while you're really trying, it's not actually a solution. In fact, it may be leading you to feel crazy around food and gain weight.

It's also very important to note that diet rules aren't the same as healthy habits. Diet rules are blamey and shamey. And they're all about weight control. Many diet rules require you to compromise your wellbeing to stick to them, leading to feelings of guilt and deprivation. Or you're asked to cut out whole food groups or skip your social life in order to stick to them. On the other hand, healthy habits support you to feel good in your body. Many healthy habits may also have a natural flow-on effect to your weight, but weight loss isn't the goal. Nor is it the metric for measuring success. Healthy habits don't make you feel guilty, nor do they make you feel like you've fallen off the bandwagon when you deviate off course. A healthy habit or healthy belief system won't demonise certain food groups or nutrients either. And after you've eaten more than you planned after a long weekend or holiday, you can return to the comfort of your healthy habits instead of falling back into the allure of a detox or diet.

Ditching diet rules

Choosing what to make for dinner every night until you die is hard enough. Percolating diet rules only take real health further out of reach. Let's make space by decluttering diet rules so that they don't make feeling good in your body even harder.

Shameless plug: my Back to Basics app is designed to take out the guesswork and help you be healthy without dieting.

✎ Challenge your diet rules

1. **Review your list of 'Diet Rules'**

   Look back at the diet rules you wrote down (see page 36) and pick one to challenge. Prioritise the rules that are having the greatest impact on your life. Alternatively, you can start with the easiest-to-destroy diet rule first. You may also want to enlist the help of a specialist non-diet dietitian to help you (in fact, I would highly recommend it).

2. **Challenge your belief**

   A diet rule isn't a fact. There are many ways to be healthy. For example, a Danish diet is different from a Mediterranean diet and yet both can be considered healthy approaches. Just because a diet book has given you certain rules, it doesn't mean that it is the only way (or even a viable way) for you. You can choose whether or not it's something you subscribe to.

   Ask yourself:
   * When and where did you first learn about this diet rule?
   * Where did this diet rule originate from? Who invented it?
   * Who has profited by this diet rule existing?
   * How did people live before this diet rule existed? Were they better or worse off?
   * Are there examples of people living healthily and happily without this diet rule?
   * Is there any research or evidence that contradicts this rule?

3. **Challenge your behaviour**

   This step involves physically challenging your diet rule, slowly stretching your comfort zone until it is no longer one of your beliefs. For example, if you believe certain fruits are fattening, you might write a list of those fruits and buy a new one each week, integrating it into your diet so that it feels less scary; if your diet rule is that you can't go back for a second helping even if you're hungry, then you could challenge this rule by giving yourself permission to dish up more food depending on your hunger using the hunger scale (see page 148) as a guide; if your diet rules make you worry that a sandwich has too many carbs, you can make or order a sandwich for lunch.

Ask yourself:

* ✻ How does this food or way of eating make me feel?
* ✻ Do I enjoy this food? Do I enjoy this different way of eating?
* ✻ What would happen if I ate this food more often?

4. **Repeat steps 1–3 with another rule on your list.**

✎ An example

1. **Diet rule:** 'pasta is bad for me'

2. **Challenge your belief**
    * ✻ **When did you first learn about this rule?** I was about 13 when I started counting points and following meal plans.
    * ✻ **Where did this diet rule originate from? Who invented it?** It probably started around the time the Atkins diet was popular.
    * ✻ **Who has profited by this diet rule existing?** The person who wrote that book would have earned a lot of money from selling the idea. Magazines would sell more copies by sharing it.
    * ✻ **Are there people who live healthily and happily without following this rule? Is there any research or evidence that contradicts this rule?** The Institute of Research analysed the diets of 23,000 Italians.[28] Not only did they find that there wasn't a correlation between eating pasta and weight gain, but they found people who ate pasta tended to weigh less.
    * ✻ **How did people live before this diet rule existed?** Lots of people around the world eat pasta and are also healthy. Pasta isn't bad or fattening. It's just a story I've been told. It's one way of eating and there are lots of ways to eat and be healthy.

3. **Challenge the behaviour**
    Make yourself some tasty pasta to eat. Or go out to a delicious Italian joint in town. While eating pasta, remind yourself, 'I am allowed to eat pasta.' Notice how the pasta makes your body feel. How much pasta did you eat before you felt satisfied or full? Was the experience what you expected?

You haven't failed at diets. Diets have failed you.

Tune out nutrition noise and tune into your body

By challenging a diet rule, you gain crucial insights into what makes your body feel good – and what doesn't. After all (and this is important) there are tonnes of ways to be healthy. Building health is a process of learning what works for your body. Noticing how certain foods or activities make you feel is a pretty reliable system for identifying what is good for your unique body, lifestyle and needs. Some people don't feel amazing after having gluten, but most people can eat it and feel fine. Others prefer how satisfied they feel with full-cream milk, while it makes other people feel sick.

Your body has a vested interest in keeping you safe, alive and thriving so it's worth trusting it a bit more, yeah?

Finding your version of health is about focusing on the way foods make you feel. It's tuning out of the nutrition noise, listening less to what other people think and instead trusting your body's innate intelligence. Bloating, fatigue or crankiness could show you're not living your shiniest life, while more energy, regular bowel movements, falling asleep easily and feeling comfortable after eating can be clues you're doing things your body likes.

If you discover you actually don't like pasta or you don't feel fab after having a second helping, how very lovely to know! Now, instead of believing 'pasta is bad for me', you think, 'I can eat pasta when I want, but I choose not to eat it because I don't love how it makes me feel'. Can you believe how different that is? Suddenly, there is choice. Eating a certain way no longer feels like a punishment or something that you have to do, that requires willpower to enforce. Rather, it's a preference. A decision. It's the difference between being externally motivated and internally motivated. And it's game-changing stuff.

Healthy habits

* ✷ are about feeling good
* ✷ support your mental and physical health
* ✷ focus on enjoyment and balance
* ✷ are timeless
* ✷ make your life better
* ✷ are a choice

Diet rules

* are about weighing less
* may require you to sacrifice your physical and mental health
* are often unsustainable
* are trend-based
* often contradict one another
* feel like a chore or punishment

Still can't tell if you're on a diet? Don't worry, I've got your back. Take my free quiz to find out if you're accidentally dieting by visiting my website at *lyndicohen.com/bookresources*.

Essential takeaways

* Dieting is seriously bad for your health. Statistically, dieting leads to weight gain, not weight loss. It leads to increased cravings and food obsession, makes you desire more food, and is awful for your self-worth.
* Many seriously wonderful people are accidentally dieting by subscribing to a long list of diet rules. Diet rules make healthy eating and consistent exercise harder.
* Becoming aware of your diet rules is a crucial step to creating a healthy relationship with food. Once you're aware of your diet rules, you can begin to challenge them one by one, so that they lose power of you.
* One strategy to do this is to use logic and rational thinking to challenge the idea that your food beliefs are 'fact'. Another strategy is to challenge yourself to go against what the diet rule tells you, thus helping to form a new behaviour.

Chapter 2.

Get off the diet rollercoaster

You're smart. You already know that health is a marathon, not a sprint. But, at times, you've been so blinded by the desire to lose weight, so motivated to break free from that 'ick' feeling in your body, that you go from never exercising to signing up for a 5 am boot-camp (even though you hate circuit training). Or you return to a weight-loss method that once worked for you, only to find you can no longer stick to it, a common state called diet burnout. And so you oscillate from daily takeaway and boozy weekends to kale salads and nightly meditation.

This is the all-too-familiar diet rollercoaster. In this chapter, we'll talk about the things that keep you stuck on the diet rollercoaster, and how to get off at the next stop and return to solid ground.

Like me (and probably you as well), my client Katie had spent her whole life dieting. So by the time she arrived at our first appointment she'd been trapped in the all-or-nothing cycle with food and her weight for many of her 36 years. And now, she was finally done.

She leaned towards me, removed her reading glasses, and explained in a clear, calm voice, 'Lyndi, I'm not expecting perfection, but I would love to be able to stop swinging from "being good" to eating to the point of being uncomfortable.' I knew exactly what she was talking about. Then she added, 'I'd also love to be able to eat a biscuit or a piece of chocolate without being driven to finish the packet. I've been doing that my whole life and it's not working for me.'

She was right. And if you can relate to one or more of the following, you can probably benefit from making a mindset shift, too.

* I eat really well during the week but I blow out on the weekend.
* I try to be 'good' or undereat when I've eaten something 'bad'.
* Seeing a number on the scale that I did not want makes me feel like I've failed.
* I have tried quitting sugar/carbs only to binge on them later.
* I feel like nothing I do is good enough.
* If I start eating unhealthily, I think, 'I may as well keeping going, finish the packet and start fresh tomorrow.'
* I'm either really good or eating ice cream straight from the tub. There's no in-between.

Sound familiar? This is what I call an 'all-or-nothing' approach. Often, uttering words like 'always', 'never' or 'have to' will be a good hint that you're stuck in this unhelpful mindset. Like a pendulum at full length, you're swinging so fast from one extreme to the other that you can never get to that restful place in the middle.

Diet burnout

If you're a frequent-flyer dieter, you might have noticed this frustrating thing happening. Each dieting attempt has become less effective than the one before. When you first started dieting, you could stick to the plan for a while. Maybe you even had quite a bit of success and longevity. You lost weight like you wanted to, you felt great and everyone told you what a wonderful higher-level, saintly being you were. But with each subsequent diet pursuit, you've become less able to stick to diet rules, structured eating or gruelling exercise.

And now, even after you've gone back to the original plan, app or program that once worked, things have changed. You just can't do it anymore! You now barely last a few hours or days of trying to be 'good' before you end up crouching in the pantry scavenging for anything with a calorie. Perhaps you're becoming less tolerant of the bullshit? Possibly. (I hope so!) You're probably experiencing diet burnout.

While diet burnout is frustrating, it's actually driven by the inbuilt protective mechanism we know as starvation mode. You start a diet but, as your body protests the deprivation and slows your metabolism, the motivation quickly dissolves into eff all. Hunger increases, weight loss slows or you gain weight even though you are eating the exact same food. Or you get flung into a cycle of good–bad eating, propelled by guilt and shame.

Do you have diet burnout?
Here are some quick ways to know if you're in the land of diet burnout:

* You can only stick to a diet for a few hours, days or weeks.
* You are constantly starting from scratch.
* You would love to get healthier but you feel paralysed to do anything differently.

* When you think about all the things you have to do to get to your goal weight, you feel overwhelmed and end up doing nothing.
* You feel disheartened and desperate about your weight yet you feel stuck, or you are – frustratingly – gaining weight.
* Your weight feels like a problem that's holding you back.

Why the hate–hate relationship? Your body associates dieting with being unsafe, a stressful state where food is scarce. So unfortunately, you can't simply 'try harder' or recruit more willpower. While you think your conscious brain (free will and all that jazz) is in control, your unconscious has a vested interest in keeping you safe. Which means fed. And nourished. It'll almost always pick binge or overeating over starvation any day of the week.

The only way to recover from diet burnout is to stop dieting. To finally accept that even though you once lost weight with group weigh-ins and calculating calories, it doesn't mean you will lose weight again. But that is not to say there is no hope and that you should give up on health efforts. On the contrary, there are many pathways one can take to be healthier, and I am offering an alternative direction with the insights presented in this book.

The willpower fallacy

It's hard to shake the feeling that if you just 'tried harder' or 'had more willpower' you'd be able to lose weight. Things would be different! After all, you've seen friends or colleagues who've shed kilos or you've run into an old acquaintance who is now much slimmer. See! It can be done.

Part of the reason you're stuck on the diet rollercoaster is that you believe getting healthy means losing weight (it doesn't) and you are relying on willpower to help you make changes. Willpower is good for tasks like getting through a boring presentation or smiling when your mother-in-law asks why you don't clean your house more often. But willpower is completely unreliable, like that flaky friend who constantly cancels on you, or who is too busy flirting with the bar staff when you need a wingperson.

This is the willpower fallacy. We convince ourselves that sticking to a diet is as simple as trying hard enough. Just because it occasionally happens for some people, we assume it should be possible for us as well. But relying on willpower to be healthy is like relying on your cat to wake you up for an important meeting. Yes, it MAY happen . . . but it's very unlikely, and there are much better solutions.

It can be quite helpful to think of willpower like a computer's RAM. When you have too many tabs open, the computer gets over-loaded. Struggling to keep up with the demands and requests, the whole system freezes. A spinning wheel appears . . . Human willpower is much the same. This is why willpower might be enough to get you started on a health journey, but it's not enough to keep you firmly planted in healthy habits over the long term.

Keep in mind that eating healthily and exercising isn't the only thing that you rely on willpower for. Simply getting through your day will burn through precious willpower. Each task, from making your bed to putting away your folded laundry, uses another little byte of your willpower RAM.

The mistake most people make is relying on willpower to lose weight or get healthy and to stay there. Depending on it over the long term. Wearing it thin, resulting in it failing you. When you most need it, it feels like your willpower has popped off early to enjoy happy hour while you ravage the fridge.

Stop relying on willpower

When you reach a weight-loss plateau your body may have activated starvation mode, so further restricting food by more intense dieting may only serve to boost your appetite and slow your metabolism.

This could explain why it's easier to stick to your diet earlier in the day, lapping up your chia pudding and chowing down a tasteless salad for lunch, but you when you get home in the afternoon, fatigued (and maybe stressed, emotional or both), your willpower leaves you quicker than you can say, 'Where are the damn chocolate biscuits?'

In Part 2 of this book, I'll introduce you to the hierarchy of healthy habits, along with essential and doable skills so that you can reduce your dependence on willpower and find more consistency with your health.

Health-kick highs and the health pendulum

If dieting is a rollercoaster ride, what we want is a nice smooth road to better health. We need balance. Existing on salad alone and living at the gym isn't 'balance'. And nor is getting sloshed on boxed wine each week and ordering enough takeaway to fund the delivery driver's upcoming wedding in Bali.

I've seen this happen with tonnes of clients. They find themselves in a 'health-kick high'. It's the buzz you get when you start doing healthy things. It can feel great to finally have broken free from the inertia of diet burnout. There's a goal weight in mind and you're going after it. You're liking the person you are while you're doing these things. You're optimistic that this could be the new you!

Feeling motivated and renewed, you sign up to a sparkly gym and buy expensive superfoods. The high you get from being on a health kick convinces you to take on a tonne of new habits in one go. This is how, if you're not mindful of it, the health-kick high can lead to a major swing in the health pendulum.

So we adopt all the habits we want, all at the same time. We go from partying too much to alcohol-free living. From not exercising much at all to early mornings at daily HIIT classes. From eating out often to following intense low-carb diets. We all know balance is the key, but when we're feeling blah in our bodies, having a bad body-image moment, we're more likely to adopt too many habits all at once. Not only that, we are also more likely to adopt extreme, unsustainable goals.

The biggest mistake we make is to go too hard, too fast. It's understandable that we do this. We want to feel better NOW. We are propelled by hating how we look or feeling crummy after seeing a photo in which we hate how we looked. We believe the quicker we get this done while motivation is high, the faster we'll get there.

One of the major flaws with the health-kick high is that it doesn't last, just like a drug-induced high. With time, your willpower reserves deplete, the initial momentum wanes (especially if you hit a weight-loss plateau), you have a week of less-than-perfect eating or you injure yourself. Any setback can break the spell. Even though it feels so good to be in it, it's not a long-term strategy for health.

In your life, there will naturally be moments when you're healthier. And times when you do less healthy things. That's normal and all part of living a healthy life. Someone who has never dieted before instinctually understands this. When they eat more than they usually do, like when they're on holiday, they don't try to compensate by skipping meals or going on a diet once they get back home. They don't vow to 'be good', cut out carbs or stay in their room while the breakfast buffet is on. Instead, when they get home, they simply go back to living their life as normal. As a result, they come right back to 'balance'. Soon, equilibrium has been restored.

But for us dieters, it's different. Because we have those pain-in-the-ass diet rules, we feel immense guilt for deviating away from how we think we should be eating. The script in a dieter's brain is far less forgiving. It says, 'You messed up, you have to fix this.' Fuelled by an unnecessary sense of failure, you overcorrect and overcompensate for what you perceive as 'bad' behaviour.

It's important to realise that beating yourself up for going a little wild on the weekend doesn't help you to be healthier.[1] It can actually drive you further away from balance. When guilt kicks in on Sunday evening, instead of waking up on Monday morning and moving on with your life as usual, intense self-blame may convince you to double down on your weight-loss efforts in order to undo the long-lunching, cocktails and cheeseboard. And so you swing the health pendulum into 'strict' or 'clean eating' territory. You throw yourself into a weight-loss pursuit, or skip meals. You overcorrect for something that didn't need correcting.

Each time you overcompensate for 'bad' eating, the health pendulum tends to swing even more intensely away from health.

You may end up with increased cravings, intense hunger and feeling deprived. And so, by the following weekend you feel the need to let loose after being so 'good' all week. And the cycle continues. Each time this happens, you get further away from health, away from balance.

Further from your goal. And this pendulum continues to swing, never allowing you to gently sway in the middle where balance exists. Finding a bit more balance is the goal.

I'm not going to suggest you give up on your hangouts with your besties or trips to the vineyard (that's a sure-fire way to suck joy out of life). The key to breaking this viciously swinging pendulum? Breaking up with guilt; noticing it and roadblocking it before it triggers another extreme. Guilt might look like lying in bed at night, upset with yourself for eating the leftover sandwich crusts from your preschooler's lunch box or for eating the entire box of chocolates you were meant to sell for charity; or guilt might turn up to ruin your mood when you skip a day or a week of workouts, resulting in you feeling like a failure.

Guilt is often the thing that drives the pendulum to swing to the extremes, along with all those noisy diet rules. So work on noticing when guilt is winding you up and learn to forgive yourself, not punish yourself. In Part 2, we'll also be focusing on how to build strong, healthy habits that feel enjoyable and doable. When you notice the temptation to swing to an extreme, this will be the thing you can always come back to.

Shifting towards balance

Here's an idea. What if there is nothing wrong with eating a bit healthier during the week and indulging a little on the weekend? Like when you get back from holidays and you suddenly crave home-cooked, lighter meals again, there's a certain balance that comes from relaxing around food and having fun.

Of course, if the divide between your weekend and weekday eating feels like a giant leap, there are things you can do so that it's less extreme.

✱ Relaxing how you eat during the week with fewer diet rules will certainly help soften the difference in your eating and exercising patterns between a weekday and a weekend.
✱ Alcohol is an important thing to consider, too. There are a whole bunch of people who choose to be alcohol-free (which is fab). There are also month-long campaigns encouraging us to give up alcohol completely, and if you find laying off alcohol temporarily

helps you drink less in the long term, I'm all for it. But the idea of committing to temporary abstinence, only to binge drink when the restrictions are lifted, feels like just another pendulum swing. What if the aim is rather to drink a little less rather than going cold turkey, which feels like bandaid fix instead of a real solution? Alternating alcoholic drinks with a glass of water is a smart thing to do as it can help you drink less and reduce the effects of a hangover. Changing the way you catch up with friends – suggesting a walk or picnic sometimes instead of a night out, or brunch instead of dinner – can also help.

✱ When doing healthy stuff doesn't feel like a punishment or chore, you might find you're happy to do these things on the weekend as well. We'll talk about this more in Part 2.

✱ Using the hierarchy of healthy habits (see Chapter 4) can help you find more balance by prioritising the stuff that matters the most, rather than wasting precious willpower 'trying to be good'.

✎ What to do when you notice the urge to diet

1. Notice guilt (without judgement)

Becoming aware of guilt is the first step. After all, guilt is the petrol that fuels dieting attempts and leads to extreme pendulum swings in health. For example, are you lying in bed at night doing mental arithmetic to work out if you've been 'good' or 'bad' that day? This may be a sign that guilt has turned up.

2. Forgive yourself

You really don't need to eat perfectly to be healthy. Let me repeat that again. You don't need to eat perfectly to be healthy. Keep this statement with you in your back pocket, so when you get a whiff of guilt, you can remind yourself of this important statement. You probably already know that this is true, but reminding yourself of it often may help prevent those dreaded and mightily unhelpful feelings of guilt, shame, regret and anger that can follow eating more than we planned, or not eating perfectly.

3. **Reframe your guilt**

Often, we feel guilt when our behaviour goes against the set of 'rules' we've been taught about how things 'should' be. But what if the very blueprint for what you 'should' be doing is wrong? Instead of seeing guilt as a sign of your weakness, consider that it's actually a signpost that you need to challenge the 'rules' and adopt better, more realistic thinking around food and health.

Essential takeaways

* You're not imagining it. Each dieting attempt is becoming less effective due to diet burnout. The only way to recover from diet burnout is to stop dieting.
* There are many ways to be healthy. Letting go of dieting may enable you to be able to forge a new and better way forward.
* Believing that willpower is the solution to help you get healthy and stay there sets you up for all-or-nothing living. This is the willpower fallacy. If you want to be more consistently healthy, you need to stop relying on willpower.
* Overcompensating for eating more than we planned can lead the health pendulum to swing from very unhealthy to obsessively healthy. Finding balance is key to long-term health.
* Food guilt fuels the health pendulum to swing to extremes. Breaking up with guilt by noticing when it happens and adjusting your self-talk is key.

Chapter 3.

The BMI is BS (and how to actually measure health)

Being healthy has become synonymous with being thin. As a result, it's hard to distinguish the difference between health advice and weight-loss advice. This is a problem, because a lot of weight-loss advice is really (and scarily) eating-disorder advice in disguise. Just consider how most diets require you to sacrifice your wellbeing or give up your social life in the pursuit of weighing less.

In our current world, sadly, it's more acceptable to have an eating disorder than to exist in a larger body. As we've learned, we're shamed for being the 'wrong weight' and told to diet. Diet companies and influencers perpetuate the problem, spruiking wellness fads for their profit; magazines publicly shame people about their bodies, while simultaneously paying lip service to the body positive movement. We're told to 'burn more, eat less'; to work to improve how we look yet somehow love our bodies. Meanwhile, mannequins in stores are so thin that even the smallest size clothes need to be pinned onto them. As a result, our self-worth is often determined by how much we weigh.

We've been told that weight is an essential metric for measuring health. Beauty ideals have infiltrated health and it's bad news for our wellbeing. There's a lot to blame for this phenomenon. Let's explore some of the key myths many of us have been led to believe.

The BMI and other weight myths

Myth #1: BMI is a measure of health

There are plenty of slim people with so-called perfect bodies who wake up fatigued, grumpy and losing their hair from not having enough nutrients in their diet. And others who smoke, drink a lot of alcohol, eat mostly takeaway. But because they are slim, the world assumes they are healthier than someone who is in a larger body who exercises regularly, eats a wholesome diet and likes themselves. If someone is in a larger body, we assume they are unhealthy regardless of how many vegies they eat or whether they go to bed at peace with themselves.

Old-school nutrition will tell you that you need to fall within the 'normal' weight range according to your Body Mass Index (BMI) to be considered healthy. But if you are looking for the answer to 'how healthy am I?', scrap the BMI. What fires me up more than any other thing when it comes to health is how many scientifically incorrect myths are peddled as fact.

The BMI is perhaps one of the most pervasive myths there is. An idea that has been adopted as fact, even though it's intrinsically flawed. So it's time for a quick history lesson. The BMI was invented by a statistician, not a medical professional. Nearly 200 years ago, Adolphe Quetelet developed a simple equation using only height and weight to get a better idea of health trends in a large population.[1] He never intended the BMI to be used to measure an individual's health. But because it was convenient, non-intrusive and could be used for anyone with a body, the BMI was adopted as an easy and inexpensive way for doctors to assess a patient's weight.

BMI doesn't take into account muscle mass, diet quality, mental wellness, sleep quality, fitness or any other metric.[2] Some people may fall within a 'healthy weight range' according to the BMI but have a non-ideal body fat percentage, while those with greater muscle mass may appear to be overweight or obese using the BMI. There are many scientifically valid ways to measure health, such as checking in on your blood pressure, cholesterol levels, fitness or blood sugar levels. When looking at a patient's health, the entire person needs to be considered. Some health care professionals can get preoccupied with BMI, failing to address the patient's concerns or assuming this number automatically indicates poor health. And that's just wrong.

My friends, we've been lied to. Some of the lies are easy to spot; for example, most of us have wised up to the fact that detox teas and appetite-suppressing lollipops are not responsible for the Kardashians' bodies. We're switching off from this messaging on social media.

Myth #2: It's always better to weigh less

There is a point when excess body weight can place a strain on the body. When joints strain from the extra load. When your body can't produce enough insulin for its needs. The fat to be mindful of is visceral fat that collects around your core organs. It's this fat that can increase your risk of heart disease, cancer and diabetes.[3] But the point when a body reaches this zone isn't always measurable by the BMI.

There's so much noise about the perils of excess weight, but it's important to remember that a certain amount of fat on your body is healthy for you. Fat is essential for our bodies to function, while also providing cushioning for injury prevention and a layer of insulation to keep us warm. If you become sick, having fat can help with recovery and ensure you've got the energy reserves to fight it off.

There is a protective role of obesity that gets swept under the scientific rug. Older people or those with several chronic conditions who are obese fare better than those who are slim.[4] They have a lower mortality (death) rate. And obesity may help curb the disease state or assist in recovery. In cancer patients, obesity seems to be linked with smaller tumour size, less aggressive forms of cancers and less progressed stages of the disease.[5] And research has shown better survival rates among those who are obese and have chronic heart failure, chronic obstructive pulmonary disease (COPD), or have a stroke and end up in intensive care.[6] The research points to better survival rates after some surgeries and fewer post-surgical complications.

Nutrition professionals are taught this in university. If sick people, especially older folks, weigh a bit more it can be protective. Those who are skinny don't do as well, we're told. People in larger bodies have protective energy reserves to help them fight illness. And perhaps their hormones fire differently thanks to the extra padding.

Sounds confusing? That's because it is. It goes against everything we're ever told: that 'fat is bad'. In fact, scientists – those very cool nerds who fuel us with valuable information – are themselves perplexed. They can't rationalise what the research is saying, so they just called it 'the obesity paradox'.

But it's not actually a paradox. What if obesity – as defined by the BMI – isn't as evil as we've been told? I'm not promoting obesity by saying this. I'm challenging the idea, the pervasive thinking that thinner is always better, that a 'healthy BMI' is automatically an indication of better wellness, when, clearly, the research says otherwise. I'm against the idea that just because someone has a BMI above 25, it automatically means they are unhealthy. There are many ways to scientifically measure health and BMI isn't a reliable method.

Body fat percentage

The current beauty ideal and fitness culture has sold us the belief that a low body-fat percentage is desirable. But in reality, crazily unfun and unhealthy things happen to your body when your fat drops below its happy spot. Women need a certain body fat percentage in order for our hormones to function well. Losing too much fat can mean your period stops, which is often a warning signal from your body. It's healthy to have some fat on your body.

Myth #3: Weight loss is the only way to get healthy

Have you ever had the experience of going to your doctor to explain something you need sorted, only for your symptoms to be ignored because the doctor has one thing on their mind: weight loss. While you try to explain your crippling anxiety or speak of a recurring headache, they tell you that it's time to lose weight, as though you haven't tried. Little do they know how much you've tried!

Your doctor might not be across this just yet, but get this: moderate to high levels of exercise can markedly reduce or eliminate the mortality risk you so often hear is linked to obesity.[7] The truth is, weight loss isn't consistently linked with increasing your lifespan. Exercising (regardless of whether or not you lose weight) can positively impact your heart health, helping those oh-so important biomarkers (think blood pressure, cholesterol, heart rate) improve.[8] This boost to heart wellbeing can be equivalent to a weight-loss program, though such programs are often touted as the only solution.

Here's the last bit of important info to come from this research. Weight cycling – that is, when you lose weight and regain it repetitively (sound familiar?) – isn't great for you. In fact, it may be worse for your health than simply existing in a larger 'overweight' body.[9] Weight cycling may be linked with higher mortality rates.[10] And higher rates of depressive symptoms.[11] That's the punishment for trying to be good.

And yet, weight-loss diets are often pushed as the only option. Beyond that, exercise with weight loss as the end goal is pushed at you. Exercising for weight loss? You've tried it. Not fun. Gruelling. Disappointing and discouraging when the weight doesn't come off. Especially tricky when you acknowledge that some types of exercise may increase your hunger levels too.[12] But exercising for enjoyment? To look after your heart health, have more energy, support your mood and brain health, all while doing things you enjoy? It can be quite lovely, indeed.

Some doctors, like the one I saw during the height of my eating disorder, are accidentally dishing out diet advice. Why are our doctors still suggesting we start a diet even though they've been shown to be ineffective?[13] Good question. Our doctors want the best for us. They're good people, I'm convinced of it. But they're not immune to the compelling allure of diets and years of believing the BMI is fact.

If your doctor keeps pushing weight loss, try these phrases:

* Please don't weigh me unless it's medically necessary (if needed, you can request a 'blind weigh-in' where they know the number, but it's not something you need to be told).
* Given the short time we have together, I'd like to focus on . . .
* I really have tried to lose weight multiple times, with very dedicated efforts. Given that diets have an exceptionally low success rate, I'd like to focus on changes that do have strong evidence to support them.
* I have a history of disordered eating/an eating disorder. Weight-loss advice isn't suitable for me.
* What advice would you give to someone thin who was in the same situation?

Myth #4: Your goal weight is your healthy weight

Fact: The *Titanic* was longer than a toothpick.

Also fact: Your healthy weight might not be the same as your goal weight.

For my wedding day, I got down to my goal weight. I'd lost enough weight that my dress kinda hung off me and my boobs were deflated (a symptom of stress and probably feeling the pressure to look the part). Yet, according to my BMI, I was in the middle of the healthy weight range for my height. Everyone told me how amazing I looked. But was I living my healthiest life? No. I was exercising too much, not eating enough and lying in bed for hours at night with insomnia caused by anxiety. But to the outside world, everyone would have considered this goal weight my healthy weight.

Your healthy weight (for right now) is probably not the same weight as on your wedding day or the same as your healthy weight in high school. It might be for some, but it probably isn't for most of us. Newsflash! Your body and weight is allowed to change throughout your life.

How much should I weigh? Trust me, you can be healthy without using an ideal weight calculator. At your healthy weight, you have plenty of energy, your hormones are balanced, your mood is lifted. Your body wants that for you.

Sadly, I still remember thinking I should have lost more weight. These unattainable beauty standards twist us into never feeling thin enough.

Myth #5: Extreme, fast weight loss is aspirational

There are many things to hate about before-and-after photos. The way they show a sad, shadowy person in the first shot followed by a beaming 'after' photo. The way they don't actually show what happens AFTER the after photo was taken. Did that person regain the weight, as so many people do? That's conveniently hidden. But perhaps the thing I find hardest to handle is how often extreme timelines are attached to the person's weight loss 'transformation'.

* Andrew lost three kilos [7 lb] in one week using our service!
* Evelyn shed half her weight in six months.
* Kaelee went down four dress sizes in 12 weeks.

Making rapid weight loss aspirational is incredibly misleading and damaging. These 'inspiring transformations' glorify extreme action. Undereating and overexercising; fasting-style diets or cutting out whole food groups; weighing out your food. If we were a little more honest with ourselves, we'd look at our past failed diet attempts and recognise that every diet we've tried before has failed us. Why would this one suddenly be different?

It's optimism bias in action: the mistaken belief that we're more likely to reach a positive outcome.

Myth #6: Losing weight will stop you hating your body

Perhaps you've been at this point or you're there now? You feel deeply uncomfortable in your clothes, that roll of fat that creeps over the top of your jeans is a constant niggle, making you feel like you need to fluff your T-shirt over and over again to prevent others from noticing it. Or there's a special event coming up and you don't have anything to wear, or you hate how you look in photographs. The 'ick' we feel in our bodies and the shame we carry around with our weight may propel us into another diet.

The desire to lose weight is so strong and not to be underestimated when you recognise it's tied to your very sense of self-worth. You convince yourself that 'this time will be different' even though it's always ended the same way. But focusing on weight loss can often be the very thing setting you up for failure.

Here are some reasons why you shouldn't focus on weight loss as a way to feel better about your body:

* When you hit a weight-loss plateau, you lose motivation when you don't see the scale moving. When weight loss is the metric for how you measure self-worth, it's a natural reaction.
* Striving to lose weight may activate starvation mode, which trips up weight-loss effort.
* When you finally reach your goal weight, you'll think you've reached your destination. You'll go back to the way you lived before, leading to weight regain (and the cycle repeats).
* It's exhausting hating your body. You miss the things you had to cut out of your diet or life. You miss bread or pasta. You miss eating when you want and socialising with friends or sleeping in.
* As you lose weight, you feel less uncomfortable in your body, reducing the 'ick' sensation that is propelling you to obsessively eat 'clean' or go to the gym. The motivation wanes.

If you're like most people and regain weight following a diet, the self-hatred can be overwhelming and life-limiting. When you run into people, they no longer comment on your weight so you assume they must think you've 'let yourself go'. You wonder if they're talking about you behind your back. You hide from going out until you can lose the weight again. You try to squeeze into your skinny clothes, which only ends up making you hate your body more. You emotionally eat to deal with all of this discomfort and heartbreak, completely overwhelmed by the idea of having to do it all over again, yet another time.

You can't hate yourself into a version of yourself that you love.

Turns out, like your university 'friend' who ditched you the moment they spotted someone cooler, self-loathing is pretty flaky. Hating your body and striving for weight loss as the solution doesn't bring long-term motivation. Making weight loss the goal makes you more susceptible to inevitable speed bumps and humps, as my client Jessie recognised: 'I'm 41 years old and I realise I've been putting a tonne of pressure on myself to lose weight so I remain healthy. In trying to do so, I've made the problem so much bigger than it really is.'

The lack of a contingency plan

Many lovely humans say with shiny optimism, 'I'll first lose the weight and then I'll make a plan for keeping it off.' That's the point where I try my darndest not to go squinty-eyed or tilt my head like a parrot. You see, it's not logical to aim to lose weight without a plan for how you're going to keep it off. Or even requiring two separate plans all together – one for the actual weight-loss process and then a second, elusive maintenance plan that's somehow meant to keep it off for good. Weight-loss advice rarely teaches you what to do once you've lost weight. What happens after you've taken the 'after' photo?

Health before weight

I'm not suggesting you disregard your health habits and give up. Instead, it's time to prioritise how your body feels and functions over what other people think of it. It's time to stop using the BMI or the number on the bathroom scale to determine whether you're progressing. The reality is that your body doesn't need to look perfect to be healthy. Let's shift the focus away from weight loss, and towards real health.

Stop actively trying to lose weight

Scary thought? But take a moment to consider: if focusing so much on weight loss has led you here, what would happen if you did precisely the opposite?

For me, shifting my focus away from weight loss and towards health was the best thing I did. Before making the leap, I calculated the risk. The worst-case scenario was that I would gain more weight and I was scared – actually terrified – of that happening, but I also realised I needed to make a change. I rationalised that years of dieting had led to unhealthy habits and deep unhappiness. So if I did the opposite, not-dieting, and stopped trying to lose weight, then there was a possibility that things would get better. I knew I didn't want to diet for the rest of my life.

So when I say I gave up dieting, a huge part of this was that I also gave up trying to actively lose weight. It took an extraordinary effort to resist the temptation to diet. Over four years, I ended up losing 20 kilograms (44 lb). This weight loss was so slow that I couldn't have measured it with a scale. Averaged out over the period, I lost 100 g (3½ oz) a week. If my goal had been to lose weight, I would have been incredibly disheartened and lost motivation when I stepped on the scale each week. I wouldn't have noticed all the other incredible progress I had made because I would have defined my success by the number on the scale. Without fast weight loss, the type you see advertised, I would have given up.

Luckily, I didn't measure my success with a scale. I measured the changes in my relationship with food and my habits, like improved sleep and reduced anxiety. I added in micro-habits, bit by bit; things that felt good and enjoyable. My mind changed for the better and, sure enough, my physical wellbeing slowly started to change with it.

I'm anti-diet. Obviously. But you've got to know that I'm not anti-weight loss. If you adopt healthy habits and you end up losing weight as a result, there's nothing wrong with that. I just don't believe in striving for weight loss as the sole motivation for how you approach your health and lifestyle. Chasing weight loss hasn't proven to be effective. As we've learned, the problem with pursuing weight loss is that having a preconceived 'goal weight' can throw you off course and muck up motivation. If the only reason you're eating healthily is so you can lose weight, then what happens after you've lost the weight? Most people return to their pre-diet eating patterns, no longer driven to weigh less.

I appreciate that you might not feel that you are currently at your healthiest weight. Maybe you feel tired, sweaty and uncomfortable in your clothes; you're desperate to shift some weight so you can feel good again. But at some point, you need to take a long-term view.

Going on a weight-loss diet is a short-term goal. It's like living in a tent instead of taking the time to build a house. Yes, building the house will take much longer, but once you've built a solid foundation, you're finally out of the all-or-nothing mindset. You get to have the lifestyle you've pined for after all these years.

Things scales can't measure

Scales will simply tell you how much your total body weighs. As a result, plenty of vital information is left out of the equation. A scale won't be able to distinguish between muscle mass (as we know muscles weigh more than fat does) or tell you what is water weight. For those who menstruate, the scale will not recognise that the weight increase just before you get your period isn't related to an uptick in total fat. And importantly, weighing yourself can't measure your happiness, fitness or health.

Stop weighing yourself

Scary, I know! But if you want a different outcome, it's time to do something different. When I was deep in my diet disorder, I put my scales in the garage. Maybe I weighed myself once a year, just out of curiosity. Because my weight wasn't the metric for my success, I wasn't as attached to what the number was.

A client of mine, 32-year-old Lori, had her own epiphany, and was brave enough to give the non-weighing thing a whirl: 'On New Year's Eve, I was doing my normal "maybe I'll give up chocolate for a year", "maybe I'll give up all sugar and processed food for a year", "maybe I'll give up dairy, carbs, sugar and wine for a year" . . . it went on. My husband, Jack, was grumbling near me (he's heard it all before) when he turned to me and said, "I wonder, could you go a whole year without weighing yourself?" It was like a light bulb! I thought to myself, if I'm not weighing myself every day, what will that change? If I don't know the dreaded number each morning, what would I do differently?

'And, amazingly, it's changed so much! Instantly, I started eating what I wanted, the amount I wanted, and was able to take in how I felt when I ate it. I gradually gave up all Coke Zero – it was making me feel bloated and sick – and just eat normal, regular simple food. The only 'rule' I have is to always eat as many vegies as I can (I can hear you cheering!) but apart from that, not weighing myself has changed so much! I've definitely lost some weight, judging by my clothes, and I'm walking more and more with my little baby in the pram, but not fussing about it.'

How to actually measure health, without scales

So if you're not measuring success by your weight, what are some other, tangible ways to track progress and wellbeing? There are a heap of things to keep an eye on if you're trying to feel energetic and your healthiest self. You will start to measure your success by how you feel, your energy levels, your blood results, your mood, and so on, and not by a number on a scale (which doesn't measure health or progress).

Ways to measure real health include:
* how much energy you have
* your blood pressure
* blood test results
* whether you like yourself and feel at peace
* you can move your body freely and easily, within your body's capabilities
* you wake up with energy
* you feel strong
* you no longer get puffed out easily

* your bowel movements
* you're progressing toward a fitness goal, such as running a specific distance or improving your flexibility
* how easily you fall asleep at night
* how many hours of quality sleep you get
* how many serves of vegetables or fruit you eat
* how happy you feel
* how often you get sick, not having swollen glands or having headaches
* when hard activities start to feel easier or you're able to do harder things as you get stronger and fitter
* when you hit your personal best or hit a new goal
* how you feel while moving your body
* your resting heart rate
* being able to do all the things you want with your body

A love note about individualism

If it's been a while since your last blood test, or if you're not feeling your flashest, making an appointment with your GP is always a good place to start. Of course, health is different for all of us, including those with different abilities. So a good GP will take into consideration the whole person instead of looking at a measure as arbitrary as height and weight.

Depending on your specific health goals, you'll need to find your own way to measure your health. My friend Eloise sure did. 'I'd always wanted to be able to do a handstand,' she told me when we caught up for dinner, 'and so I just started practising doing handstands in my bedroom. I'd film myself practising doing the handstands. Rewatching the videos, I could really see how much I was improving!'

She explained how exciting it was to be able to see herself progress towards a big goal, something completely unrelated to weight or shape, but rather movement. And something she thought was lots of fun. After months of working towards the goal, she was now holding beautiful handstands and feeling so much stronger. The change in her strength was noticeable in other areas of her life too; plus, she felt happier.

Eloise measured her health progress in a way that was unique to her, at a time in her life where that's what she wanted to achieve. In ten years' time, she may not use the same metric to track her health. Your health goals and how you measure your wellness will shift depending on the season of your life.

Another friend, Jana, explained that she measures her health based on how easily she falls asleep at night. She notices a big difference in the nights when she easily drifts into slumber compared with the nights she lies in bed fretting or feeling restless.

Since becoming a mother, my energy stores have become a major priority for me. Waking up with energy, and having the stamina to not feel depleted after a long day, is my new metric for my health. It drives me to get to sleep earlier, to exercise during the day for that essential energy and mood boost, and to say no to others instead of having to say no to myself.

A few years ago, my mood and managing my anxiety was a top priority for me. I once tracked my period for nine months with some pretty fascinating insights, which I'll talk about in more detail on page 159. Noticing how much the menstrual cycle influences mood, sleep, sex drive, bowel movements, energy, body image and more was deeply interesting to me for a time. As I grow older, no doubt the way I measure my health will shift too.

My sister-in-law Rachelle was dealing with postnatal depression and decided that a physical challenge would give her focus. She chose to attempt to swim the English Channel, swimming solo from England until she reached the shores of France. More people have climbed Mount Everest than have completed this swim! The pursuit would entail a 33 kilometre (20 mile) swim in 15°C (59°F) water, without a wetsuit, swimming past swarms of jellyfish. To make it an official crossing, she wouldn't be able to touch another boat, person or support vessel until she reached the other side.

She trained for the pursuit for three years, measuring her progress in how many training sessions she ticked off, tracking how far she could swim, her stroke rate, how cold the water was and how she was feeling mentally. She progressively worked towards a goal until one dark, cold morning she left the shore at Dover at 3 am and swam for 15 hours and 54 minutes until she made it to France. Why am I telling you this incredibly remarkable but perhaps unrelatable story? Well, Rachelle wasn't an athlete. She was a mum of three whose mental health became such a priority that she swapped tracking calories for tracking how many laps she did in a pool. And her health transformed because of it.

These are just some examples of how you can measure your own health. I'm not suggesting you take up ultramarathons or try to do handstands in your kitchen (although you can if you want to!) but the point is to find a new way of defining your health, unrelated to weight. Whether you choose to measure that progress or not is your decision. But imagine how fulfilling it would be to accomplish a goal rather than a dress size?

After all, why are we all trying to reach a goal body anyway? Isn't it so we can finally feel worthy, acceptable and good enough? From my own experience, tying these sorts of aspirations to weight loss is both unattainable and unsustainable. But I know for Rachelle or Eloise, they certainly felt much healthier and a mighty sense of accomplishment from their pursuits towards their definition of health.

Of course, it ain't easy choosing and sticking to real health goals, especially in this looks-obsessed diet world. That's why, in Part 3 of this book, we'll tackle some of the emotional hurdles that stop you focusing on health, rather than weight.

✎ How do you measure your health?

Consider your lifestyle and personal health goals.

* Of all the methods for measuring health, what is most important to you right now?
* Unrelated to weight, what is something you'd like to improve when it comes to your health? It could be energy, mental wellness or strength.
* Try to remember a time in your life when you felt brilliant health-wise. What was different about that time compared with now?
* What does your doctor or another health care professional believe is the most important way for you to measure your health right now?

A word about tracking and measuring

There's a popular expression in the business world, famously coined by mathematician and physicist Lord Kelvin. He said, 'If you can't measure it, you can't improve it.' But when it comes to health, we've become obsessed with tracking, measuring and counting. And if you're resisting the idea of tracking any measure of health, that's perfectly fine.

Dieters often have ninja-like tracking skills. We've tracked points and calories and how many grams we ate for lunch. So much so, it can be hard to deprogram yourself from mentally calculating the calories in a meal or snack. We've tracked waist circumference metrics, our dress size and weight. We've taken before-and-after photos and we've had full body scans. Did all this tracking make us obsessed or did we track because we were obsessed?

Especially in the early days of learning to free yourself from diets, you may need to abandon any form of tracking until you feel ready. Personally, I stopped any form of tracking or recording for some years.

You'll know you're ready when you feel excited to add more healthy habits in your life, when you naturally become curious about how micro-experiments will impact how you feel.

Can't lose the last few kilos?

Struggling and just can't lose the last few kilos? Do you know why it's hard to lose them?

It may be because you're not supposed to. But because society and your Instagram feed have programmed you to think that's how you 'should' look, you torture yourself to lose those last few kilos. If it feels like your body is fighting against you when you try to lose those last few kilograms, it's because your body IS fighting against you. When your weight drops below where it's meant to be, your body will fight back.

The deprivation will trigger a binge and suck you into the pendulum swings of an emotional eating cycle. Your 'dedication' will turn into fixation and obsession – and you'll become controlled by thoughts of food. And your metabolism will slow – so you'll need to eat even less and train even harder to maintain your dream weight.

What real health looks like

Going out for dinner is such fun: don't let your weight worries keep you from missing out on living your life. I like to go out for dinner with friends and family, order what I want and have a glass of wine. That's not something I'm willing to give up to look perfect in a bikini (whatever that means).

When you push your body to lose weight, you're giving up more than just calories. You miss out on life. You miss out on seeing friends. 'That sounds great!' becomes 'I'm sorry, I can't come; I need to lose weight'. You pay with your freedom, your spontaneity . . . the simple pleasures in life. Those last couple of kilos are your favourite holidays and unforgettable memories.

You give up:
* sharing laughs with your friends over a cheeseboard
* falling asleep easily, feeling satiated, happy and full
* licking the bowl after you've baked your friend a birthday cake
* eating your favourite dessert because you want to
* going to a restaurant and ordering what you want
* catching up with your best friend for dinner

These days, I won't give up these simple pleasures. I'm the healthiest I've ever been, and this is what my body looks like naturally. I'm happy with that. But I go to sleep happy with myself (without any guilt about what I ate that day) and my thoughts aren't dictated by what I'm 'allowed' to eat or whether you can see my hip bones.

If, after all we've discussed, you still find yourself resisting freedom from dieting, consider this:
* Looking good in a bikini does not mean you are healthy. Most people don't naturally have a bikini body or abs even when they are at their healthiest weight. Unfollow 'wellness' accounts that share bikini and ab shots and call it health and balance.
* When your life revolves around food and what you look like, your life and potential is limited. If you want to be successful, if you want to be great (admired, appreciated, respected), you need your

brainpower. When you starve your body, you can't think straight. When you restrict yourself, you can never be your best.

✱ Accepting your body does not mean you're giving up on yourself. It does not mean accepting that this is the best you'll ever look. Accepting your body is about knowing that you are enough as you are. It is confidence in your innate worth. And confidence, not your weight, is truly what makes you shine.

If real health is the goal (and I hope by now it is your goal!), then the hierarchy of healthy habits (see page 75) is a tool that can help us get there. It offers a new way to measure your health and take strides towards balance, without using weight as the metric for success. By focusing on habits we're focusing on health, not centimetres or kilograms. And nor are we overloading our plate with a long to-do list, either. In Part 2 of this book, you'll learn how the hierarchy of healthy habits can help prioritise real health over diet nonsense.

Essential takeaways

✱ The BMI is an outdated and unscientific measurement that can't assess your health. Nor can weighing yourself on a scale.

✱ Stop trying to lose weight (which is poor source of motivation) and start aiming to be healthy instead. Focusing on weight loss may lead to health pendulum swings and can make it challenging to adopt healthy habits that actually stick around.

✱ True health is where your hormones are balanced, your body is strong and your mood is stable. Your goal weight is the weight where you fall asleep easily, you have boundless energy and your mind is free to think about things other than macros, calories or reps at the gym.

✱ Maybe the reason you can't lose the last few kilos is because you're not supposed to. You may already be at a weight where your body feels comfortable. When you try to undercut your body's preferred weight, it may fight against you.

✱ You can't hate yourself into a version of yourself that you love.

Part 2.
A Better Way To Be Healthy

Now that you're moving away from unhelpful diet rules, food guilt and unattainable health metrics, the next step is to start adding healthy, doable habits into your life: things that help you feel fabulous in your body.

Chapter 4.

The hierarchy of healthy habits

During the 1940s, while many mental health professionals were fixated on psychopathology – trying to fix things when they went wrong in the brain – 34-year-old psychologist Abraham Maslow was deeply interested in helping people reach their potential. And so he put forward the motivational theory now commonly known as Maslow's hierarchy of needs.

Usually simplified as a five-level pyramid, Maslow's hierarchy of needs suggests that in order to reach the top level of 'self-actualisation', a human first has to fulfil their most essential needs, starting from the bottom. Once each level and its needs has been attained, the person can then move further up the pyramid towards reaching their potential.

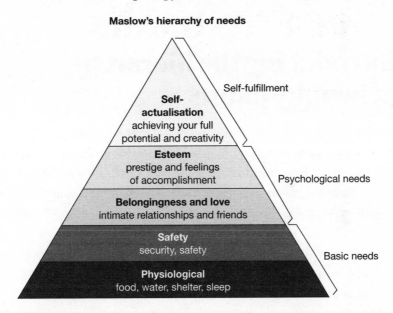

Maslow's hierarchy of needs

At the very bottom of the hierarchy are needs essential to human survival: food, water, shelter, sleep. These physiological needs must be met in order for someone to move up to the next level. After all, if you're hungry or cold, it's pretty hard to focus on much else.

The second level includes requirements for safety – things like order, stability, security and freedom from fear – while the third level relates to relationships and our need to feel connected to others, to be part of a community and have intimate relationships. Level four is focused on self-esteem, including our need to be valued, respected and recognised. Once all of these levels have been attained, Maslow suggested that you can then start to work toward self-actualisation, a fulfilled state where you may reach your potential, becoming who you were always meant to be.

Why am I telling you this? Maslow's hierarchy of needs was a game-changer in psychological fields that helped explain crucial human behaviours; like how, when you're overworked and exhausted from doing 14 loads of washing and waiting on the phone on hold for three hours, your sex drive goes mysteriously AWOL. It's understandable when you realise that your basic physiological needs, in this case rest and sleep, have gone unmet, so you're a whole lot less likely to want to play footsies with a partner at the end of another busy day.

Introducing the hierarchy of healthy habits

The hierarchy of healthy habits is a visual tool I've created, adapting Maslow's pyramid structure, to provide a new way of thinking about your health. Like learning to walk before you can run, when it comes to healthy habits some basic actions need to come first. You may dream of getting really fit, running a marathon or setting a new PB, but in order to do this, you first need to ensure you're getting enough fuel, hydration and sleep. Without these basic needs fulfilled, you're going to have a hard time accomplishing your desired goals consistently.

The hierarchy of healthy habits outlines essential habits you need to acquire to build real, sustainable health, starting with basic needs and working your way up to your ideal lifestyle. Using the hierarchy can help you identify gaps in your health, so you can focus on the most important habits first, the ones that will yield the biggest results.

In a video game, you can't start at level 500: you need to complete earlier levels, so you have the skills to negotiate that new level. Building health is much the same. You first need to acquire the skills and tick off the fundamentals of survival, before you can thrive. The problem is that most people skip the fundamentals. Or they try to jump ahead to attain a higher level without completing the groundwork first.

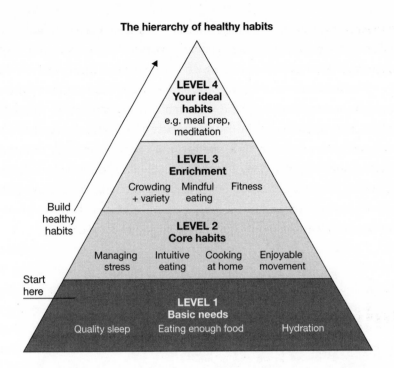

The hierarchy of healthy habits

LEVEL 4
Your ideal habits
e.g. meal prep, meditation

LEVEL 3
Enrichment
Crowding + variety   Mindful eating   Fitness

LEVEL 2
Core habits
Managing stress   Intuitive eating   Cooking at home   Enjoyable movement

LEVEL 1
Basic needs
Quality sleep   Eating enough food   Hydration

Build healthy habits

Start here

I created my hierarchy of healthy habits in response to a problem I experienced in my nutrition clinic some time ago. During a consultation with 29-year-old Maree, we'd talked about possible new habits she could adopt to achieve her goals, from cooking at home more often to practising intuitive eating. As I was still new to being a dietitian, I probably shared a bit too much information; too many strategies. I was very excited for Maree. At the end of the session, she turned and asked me, 'Oh Lyndi, I almost forgot. I wanted to ask, which is the healthiest yoghurt?' I gave her my answer, mentioning a brand I liked.

At the next follow-up session a month later, I was keen to hear what progress she'd made. 'Well, I didn't cook much, but I did swap to that new yoghurt you recommended,' she said excitedly. She felt really proud of this change, but I felt like I'd failed Maree. I'd given her too much too think about and work on. As a result, I'd overwhelmed her.

Any change is good change but, in the scheme of things, the brand of yoghurt you buy is very low in the priority list for making healthy changes. There are far more impactful things we can focus on. We often do this with nutrition: we waste precious headspace trying to count grams of sugar in salad dressing but underestimate the importance of eating more vegetables. We worry about an extra slice of bread instead of aiming to cook one more meal at home each week.

The intense amount of nutrition noise we receive can sometimes paralyse and confuse us about what really matters when it comes to health. We get distracted by the nitty-gritty of nutrition perfectionism (that tells us we can only have yoghurt if it's sugar free, dairy free and fat free), instead of staying grounded in the stuff that matters most. We waste 80 per cent of our energy trying to change the things that have 20 per cent of the impact, rather than focusing 20 per cent of our energy on things that contribute to the 80 per cent.

One of the benefits of the hierarchy is that it can help you focus on the big ticket items first, rather than getting bogged down in the stuff that's kinda helpful but doesn't really matter. It can also help take the confusion out of certain situations; for example, unsure whether to go to the gym or hit snooze after a shonky night of sleep? Knowing that sleep is the cornerstone of wellbeing can help you recognise that an extra hour of sleep may be what is really best for your body. Remind yourself that it's not a big deal, and that you'd rather use your headspace for making bigger, more important changes.

Identify habit gaps

First, let's start by identifying any gaps in your habit pyramid. Like a tower of wooden blocks with pieces pulled out, having gaps in your hierarchy of healthy habits makes you more likely to fail, especially when a turbulent, stressful period comes along. Identifying gaps, including the basic needs and habits you thought were ticked off but aren't really, is pretty important stuff; for example, if you aren't sleeping well, you're likely to experience a surge in cravings for high-energy foods such as chips, lollies and soft drink, while simultaneously having a decline in metabolism and depleted energy reserves, which results in crushingly low willpower and reduced chance of exercising. If you're consistently not eating enough because you're always on a newfangled diet, or oscillating wildly between undereating and out-of-control pantry raids, you may not be eating enough to help your body feel 'safe'. Using the hierarchy, you can address fundamental gaps that are holding you back and have a clear plan to prioritise what matters most.

The benefit of filling in those bothersome gaps is stickier habits; not feeling like you're constantly starting from scratch. Comfortable habits you can return to rather than going on another stupid diet. Oh, and your skin, sex drive, relationships, mood and immunity may also prosper from getting your basic needs met. You'll have a rock-solid foundation on which to build habits that actually stick. And you may find that some problems like struggling to commit to a consistent workout plan, or those intense 3 pm sugar cravings, may reduce.

To fill in gaps, you need to identify them. As you work through this book, create a list of any 'habit gaps' you discover in the notes app on your phone or in a notebook.

Once you're aware of the gaps, you can use the layout of the hierarchy to prioritise what to work on first, starting with any gaps in the lowest levels and working your way upward. But don't fret. You don't need to completely reach perfection in any of these habits in order to start building beyond them. Consider a new level unlocked when you're mostly or more consistently achieving these habits. The occasional poor night's sleep isn't as concerning as consistently broken slumber. Getting mostly takeaway during a particularly busy week isn't going to ruin your health if you return to cooking more at home shortly after. The aim is to simply become more consistent so these gaps no longer derail your health and wellbeing.

You can download a master worksheet from my website: lyndicohen.com/ bookresources.

Also, it's important to note that there is a bidirectional relationship between some habits, even if they exist on different levels. For example, adding enjoyable movement (Level 2) might help you get better quality sleep (an essential Level 1 need). Intuitive eating, also a Level 2 habit, might help you know if you're eating enough food for your body. Eating more fruits and vegetables might help you stay better hydrated. Reducing stress may help you sleep better, thanks to a shift in cortisol levels. This all makes sense! You may work on two different habits simultaneously; however, you can't neglect Level 1 basic needs in pursuit of habits on higher levels. Ensure the basic needs on the lower levels are getting the attention they need.

Personalising the pyramid

I'mma repeat myself as often as I need to: health isn't one-size-fits-all. Even Maslow's hierarchy of needs can't be applied for every unique human. Similarly, the hierarchy of healthy habits is a starting point, introducing a new way to think about health, enabling better prioritisation of what matters to your divine body. You can edit it so that it best serves you. If fitness is the cornerstone to your mental and physical health, so that it feels more like a core habit for you, shift it down to where it feels right for you. Live in hotel or somewhere without a kitchen so cooking is off the cards? That's all good. Leave it out or replace it with something essential for you, like meditation. You can find an editable version of the hierarchy of healthy habits on my website: *lyndicohen.com/bookresources*.

Your basic needs

Level 1 includes the basic needs you need to survive. It's fundamental that the 'basic needs' are fulfilled before trying to add in fancier and more Instagrammable health habits. And you'd be surprised how common it is to have major habit gaps starting in Level 1 (especially for ex-dieters). Let's investigate if you currently have a gap that needs mending in your basic needs.

For some people, the basics might also include taking certain medications or physical therapies, so don't forget to include those.

During stressful times, sleep, hydration and eating consistently (and enough) for your body can fall through the cracks and you may need to reassess where you're at and reprioritise basic needs.

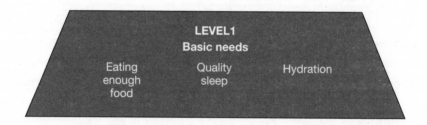

LEVEL1
Basic needs

Eating enough food

Quality sleep

Hydration

A Better Way To Be Healthy

Do you eat enough food?

You might think, 'Of course I eat enough food! My problem is that I eat TOO MUCH food.' If that's you, I want you to really tune into this section. Why? Because I often meet people (particularly those who have been dieters) who are undereating or who are making their body fear that access to food is limited or restricted.

In order to fulfil the essential need of eating enough food, your body has to trust that it has a consistent and reliable supply of energy. This means that binge eating on the weekend and 'trying to be good' during the week might trigger your body's starvation mode – something we've already discussed and we'll talk about more in Chapter 6.

Of course, not eating enough because you're subscribing to diet rules, skipping meals, overexercising or following fasting protocol can be harsh on your body. As long as your body believes food is not freely and consistently available, you'll likely find it hard to build real health. After all, it's tricky to fall asleep or concentrate when you don't have enough energy or when every thought keeps coming back to food.

How many of these apply to you? Within the past 30 days, I have . . .

* skipped meals
* become ravenously hungry
* avoided certain foods like carbs
* counted calories or macros
* followed a list of diet rules
* experienced big swings between my weekday and weekend eating
* started a new diet or decided I should try to eat less or better
* portion-controlled my meals
* experienced binge eating
* felt guilty for eating more than I planned
* forgotten to eat

Potential signs you aren't eating enough

* low energy levels
* constantly thinking about food
* hair loss or excess hair growth
* fertility issues
* feeling irritable

* sleep problems
* feeling cold when others feel warm
* constipation

Give yourself a point for each one that applies to you. The more you selected, the more likely it is that your body doesn't feel like you are eating enough. If you feel that this may be something to work on, add it to your 'habit gaps' list as the most important thing to address. We'll talk in more detail about addressing this crucial gap in Chapters 6 and 7 so that you can help your body start to trust that food is plentiful.

Do you consistently get good-quality sleep?

Sleep is the cornerstone of health. That's because sleep helps to regulate your metabolism, appetite, hormones, mood, immune system and heart health.[1] Big stuff! And yet, many of us are falling behind on the recommended seven to nine hours of uninterrupted sleep each night.

And it's not just how many hours of shut-eye you get, but the quality of your sleep that really matters. This could explain why almost 60 per cent of Australians report having sleep difficulties, such as trouble falling asleep, waking too early and not being able to fall back asleep.[2]

If you have low-quality sleep, it may mean:
* your willpower is more easily spent
* you have less energy to build healthy habits
* your mental health is placed under strain
* you're at a greater risk of developing a chronic health condition
* your appetite is boosted, with more intense cravings
* your hormones can become unbalanced

It's worth prioritising sleep before embarking on a new fitness quest or trying to consistently cook at home or eat healthier. Yet, most people overlook the importance of getting more sleep, focusing on unhelpful advice to just 'eat less and move more'. Maybe what you really need is more sleep! Is sleep a habit gap in your hierarchy of healthy habits? You may already be drowsily nodding yes. If you're unsure, you can take this quiz to find out.

1. **Do you have trouble falling asleep?**
   a. Yes, most nights.
   b. Yes, one or two times a week.
   c. Sometimes, but less than once a week.
   d. Rarely or not at all.

2. **Do you wake during your sleep and have trouble falling asleep again?**
   a. Yes, most nights.
   b. Yes, one or two times a week.
   c. Sometimes, but less than once a week.
   d Rarely or not at all.

3. **On average, how many hours of sleep have you had each night during the past 14 days?**
   a. < 5 hours
   b. > 9 hours
   c. 7–8 hours
   d. 8–9 hours

4. **How do you feel when you wake up in the morning?**
   a. Generally very tired and struggle to get out of bed.
   b. Exhausted, even though I've slept for the recommended amount of time.
   c. Reasonably well rested and don't struggle to get out of bed.
   d. Very well rested and ready to tackle the day.

5. **Do you feel drowsy or need to take naps during the day?**
   a. Yes, I am almost always drowsy and need a nap during the day.
   b. I am sometimes drowsy and need a short nap during the day.
   c. I don't generally feel drowsy or nap during the day.
   d. I never feel drowsy or have a nap during the day.

Give yourself a point each time your answer was either an *a* or a *b*. If you scored 1 or more out of 5, it's likely that sleep quality is a habit gap for you, and really worth prioritising. In Chapter 7, I'll be addressing sleep, along with all the other key healthy habits, and giving you some tangible, practical strategies for improvements. However, I strongly recommend speaking to your doctor (rather than googling solutions), because your health is worth investing in. Feeling tired all the time can be caused by a bunch of other things; it's not always just dodgy sleep. Give your favourite doctor a call if you feel tired and want to be sure it's not something else.

Are you well hydrated?

Hydration is critical to our survival and yet we often don't get enough water to replenish our system. Or we drink too much alcohol or coffee, which can have a dehydrating effect. Getting enough H_2O into your diet, whether with cups of water, herbal tea, fruits and vegetables or other food is très important for your energy levels, metabolism, concentration, mood and organ health. If you don't drink enough water, it may cause you to feel sluggish and could contribute to that 'tired all the time' feeling.[3] You may also find tuning into your hunger a little trickier because when your body isn't getting water through drinks, it may seek hydration in food form.

While I don't think a glass of water heals most ailments, ensuring you're healthily hydrated is a key and often overlooked part of looking after your body. Ultimately, it's tough to be your sparkliest, most energetic self or to tune into your hunger when you're not getting ample hydration. To see if you're getting enough, try this quick quiz.

1. **How would you describe your thirst?**
    a. I'm always thirsty.
    b. I forget to drink until I get thirsty.
    c. I drink water before I get thirsty.
    d. I drink water regularly throughout the day.

2. **The colour and smell of my urine is:**
    a. Orange, amber, strong smell.
    b. Bright yellow, noticeable smell.
    c. Pale yellow or clear, subtle smell.
    d. Clear, very pale yellow.

Give yourself a point each time your answer was either *a* or *b*. If you scored 1 or more, you may need to work on more proactively hydrating.

How did you go?

Do you have any gaps on Level 1, your basic needs for survival? If so, these are the most pressing things to work on addressing first. If you're gap-free at this point, well done. Regardless, let's continue to review Level 2 of the hierarchy to help identify if there are any gaps that need filling in your core habits.

Core habits

Unlike basic needs, the core habits found on Level 2 of the hierarchy of healthy habits are less about survival, but are also key building blocks to better health. While basic needs are the most important to address first, core habits are next in line in terms of priority. Given that intuitive eating is a helpful technique to ensure you are eating enough food, and that reducing stress and adding in enjoyable movement can aid better sleep, you may want to work on a core habit that aligns with any gaps in your basic needs.

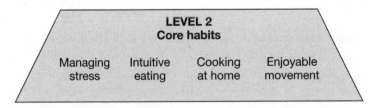

Do you have a healthy balance between stress, rest and self-care?

Some level of stress is normal, but when it impacts on your ability to function, your quality of life or important things like sleep, it's not good. High levels of stress can muck about with your hormones, mood and immune system.[4] In fact, you may drink more alcohol to help combat stress, find you emotionally eat to try to numb the discomfort or may even forget to eat. Reducing unhealthy stress levels while giving yourself the appropriate amount of self-care is the name of the game. How do you fare at this core habit right now?

1.   **How often do you take time for rest and self-care?**
   a.   I don't have time for rest or self-care.
   b.   Only once everything else on my to-do list is complete (which means it rarely happens.)
   c.   A few times a week.
   d.   As much as I need to.

2.   **How would you rate your stress level during the past 30 days?**
   a.   I've been very stressed lately.
   b.   Somewhat stressed.
   c.   Rarely stressed.
   d.   Any stress I've had has felt manageable.

3.   **During the past 30 days, how often have you been able to stay focused on the present moment?**
   a.   Never
   b.   Sometimes
   c.   Often
   d.   Almost always

4.   **During the past 30 days, how often have you felt overwhelmed?**
   a.   Almost always
   b.   Often
   c.   Rarely
   d.   Never

Give yourself a point each time your answer was either *a* or *b*. If you scored 2 or more, you may need to add managing stress to your 'habit gaps' priority list. Don't worry, the irony of adding one more thing to your to-do list during a stressful time is not lost on me! We'll cover strategies in more detail in Chapter 9 of this book.

I'd also hiiighly recommend making an appointment with a mental health-care professional such as a psychologist, counsellor or psychiatrist. I like to think of it as going to the gym for your brain; the support they offer is not just for people in crisis. Why do we proudly take care of our physical bodies but feel ashamed to get help for one of our most important organs? I've been seeing a psychologist or counsellor for more than a decade, and it's made my life less overwhelming and shinier. Oh! And I've taken anti-anxiety medication in the past as well, another hugely helpful thing I did for my mental wellbeing.

Are you an intuitive eater?

Intuitive eating is the process of tuning into your appetite. It's about eating to comfortably satisfy your body's energy requirements, and it's also about noticing and listening to how much food your body needs on any given day rather than subscribing to inflexible diet rules or portion control. In Chapter 8, I'll explain intuitive eating in far more detail along with strategies to help you eat more in sync with your body's natural hunger and fullness cues. But for now, answering these questions may help you identify if intuitive eating is missing from your hierarchy of habits.

1. **When I eat, I . . .**
   a. Don't think about what I am eating or listen to my hunger levels.
   b. Forget to tune into my hunger.
   c. Often try to tune into my hunger before eating.
   d. Almost always try to eat intuitively.

2. **After eating, I often feel . . .**
   a. Overly full
   b. Still hungry or unsatisfied
   c. Comfortably full
   d. Satisfied

3. **Before eating, I check in with my hunger . . .**
   a. Never
   b. Occasionally
   c. Often
   d. Almost always

Give yourself a point each time your answer was either an *a* or a *b*. If you scored 1 or more, then intuitive eating may be an important skill to consider working towards.

Do you regularly cook at home?

Sure, you can grab healthier choices when getting takeaway or eating out; however, cooking a healthy meal at home is in general going to be best for your health. Eating home-cooked meals can help you feel more connected to your food, support you to eat mindfully (as you may be less likely to hurriedly eat food you took time to prepare) and may also help you eat according to your hunger and fullness, knowing that food can easily be stored in an airtight container for later.

It's kinder on your budget, too.

Once you get into the habit of cooking at home more (and enjoying it, 'cause that's key), then you can progressively start cooking healthier options, crowding in more vegetables and trying new recipes. For most, cooking at home is an essential stepping stone. You can't expect to go from eating out all the time to being a meal prep–monarch overnight.

I know many people don't enjoy cooking and they're often the first to admit that they're also not the best cooks. Their dislike of cooking makes sense when you consider how failed attempts, wasted time, money, energy and a lack of compliments can make you dislike a habit. But ultimately, eating is something you are going to have to do for the rest of your life, multiple times a day. You can either spend the rest of your life avoiding and hating cooking, or you can spend a bit of time and energy to get good at it. This is a worthwhile investment that will repay you for the rest of your life. If you become better at cooking (which is not something you're born with, it's a skill you can acquire) then you may find it becomes something you start to enjoy, or at least don't hate.

1. **How often do you cook at home?**
   a. Rarely! I often get takeaway or eat out or on the go.
   b. Once or twice a week.
   c. 3–4 times a week.
   d. Five or more times a week.

2. **Do you enjoy cooking?**
   a. I'm not good at it so I don't like cooking.
   b. I try to avoid cooking.
   c. I don't mind cooking.
   d. Cooking is my vibe!

Give yourself a point each time your answer was either an *a* or a *b*. If you scored 1 or more points, cooking more at home could be added to your list of priorities (after any basic needs, of course); although if someone else in your household is responsible for the cooking, or being a person with disability means it's not something you do, then you might need to assess for yourself whether getting in the kitchen is important for you right now.

Do you engage in enjoyable movement?

Enjoyable movement is different from fitness. It includes things you do because you like how they make you feel, like going for a walk, dancing in the kitchen or stretching your body. It could include going to a yoga class, playing some casual tennis, taking the stairs or walking your dog.

Yoga may fall into enjoyable movement or fitness, depending on your approach.

Finding enjoyable movement can help give you more energy, support your mood and immune system, improve your sleep and help you feel better in your body.[5] It's not about burning calories, hitting personal bests or looking a certain way; it's rooted in feelings. While fitness is about building strength or stamina, enjoyable movement is about active living, and doing movement because you like the way it makes you feel. It doesn't have to be rigorous. You may or may not break out into a sweat. But enjoyable movement is a key ingredient to helping you develop a healthier relationship with movement (even if fitness isn't always necessarily your goal).

1. **How often do you move your body each week?**
   a. Almost never.
   b. Once or twice a week.
   c. 3–5 times a week.
   d. Every day, or almost every day.

2. **How would you describe your relationship with movement?**
   a.   I rarely ever do it because I don't really enjoy it.
   b.   I enjoy it but don't do it enough.
   c.   I'd like to do more enjoyable movement.
   d.   I prioritise movement because I enjoy it and it feels good.

Give yourself a point each time your answer was either an *a* or a *b*. If you scored 1 or more, you may want to consider adding enjoyable movement to your list. If you have an injury or are a person with disability, then you might need to decide whether this is an important habit for you. In Chapter 9, we'll dive further into enjoyable movement, why it's useful and how to go about enriching your life with it.

How did you go?

If you noticed any gaps in your core habits, add them to the 'habits gap' list, following on from any basic needs gaps. Now, it's time to move one level up, toward the enrichment habits.

Enrichment habits

While basic needs and core habits are the basis of health, these habits really are about taking your wellbeing to a new level. Once you've done the groundwork of laying a solid foundation with your basic needs and core habits, you can then start to build in enrichment habits.

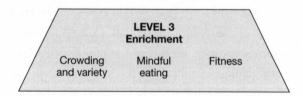

LEVEL 3
Enrichment

Crowding and variety   Mindful eating   Fitness

Do you crowd in healthy and varied ingredients?

In the past, nutrition advice has sadly been obsessed with telling us what we aren't allowed to eat. As we've seen, this can lead to increased cravings for the very foods we're trying to eat less of. This 'subtraction' approach to health, telling us to avoid sugar or eat fewer calories, hasn't worked. The new approach is all about addition, focusing on all you can eat instead of what you can't. It's about 'crowding' in more of the healthy stuff so that you naturally fill up on nutritious ingredients, without fearing certain foods or nutrients.

Balance is at the core of crowding, meaning that nothing is eliminated or forbidden. In fact, the goal is to boost variety. Eating a more varied diet has been linked with better gut health, which can have delicious flow-on effects for your mood, immune system and how you feel in your body.[6] Are you yet to add 'crowding' into your repertoire? Let's find out.

1. **When I try to eat healthily, I . . .**
   a. Focus on what I've been told avoid (carbs, sugar, fat, salt).
   b. Try to limit what I eat through a range of diet rules.
   c. Expand the list of foods I aim to eat rather than reducing the 'allowed' foods.
   d. Focus on vegetables, fruits, wholegrains, seeds and nuts. I aim for variety and try to boost my intake of the healthier stuff.

2. **How much variety do you currently get in your diet?**
   a. I stick to a meal plan irrespective of what is in season because that is what I feel comfortable eating and I don't generally try new things.
   b. I'm in a bit of a food rut as I tend to eat the same things over and over, with just a small amount of variance.
   c. I try to eat seasonally and mix it up, even if I'm not perfect at it all the time.
   d. I love eating different things and regularly change my menu based on what's in season or my latest food inspo.

Give yourself a point each time your answer was either an *a* or a *b*. If you scored 1 or more, you may want to consider practising a bit more crowding and infusing your diet with more variety. And you bet we'll chat more about how to do this soon enough, in Chapter 10.

Do you practise mindful eating?

Mindful eating is the process of tuning into the food you're eating, instead of the Kardashians. It's about being present, tasting the food and noticing how eating the meal is making you feel. The aim is not to be distracted, which means switching off the TV and sitting at the table instead of eating in the car while in traffic.

We all know mindful eating is an important thing to do. Why is it all the way up on Level 3? In order to be able to eat mindfully, you first have to address two primary barriers to mindful eating. First is eating enough food (it's hard to eat mindfully when you never feel that food is allowed) and second is the ability to eat intuitively. Regardless of whether these are still gaps for you, let's see if mindful eating is another habit to add to the 'habit gap' list.

1. **When I eat, I ...**
    a. Forget to think about what I am eating or listen to my hunger levels.
    b. Sometimes try to tune in to my hunger and think about what I am eating.
    c. Often tune in to my hunger and enjoy the process of eating.
    d. Consistently eat mindfully and intuitively.

2. **Where do you most often eat your meals?**
    a. I usually eat in front of the TV, computer or while scrolling on my phone.
    b. I usually eat on the go, sitting in the car or in a rush.
    c. I generally try to eat at the table, although this doesn't happen all the time.
    d. I almost always eat at the table, without distracting devices.

Give yourself a point each time your answer was either an *a* or *b*. If you scored 1 or more, mindful eating may need make its way onto your habit gap list.

Are you building your fitness?

Fitness includes all the things we do above and beyond basic movement. It's about building strength and stamina, flexibility, agility or trying to rev up your power. Enjoyable movement is the building block that helps you build up to fitness. But fitness isn't about looking good in a crop top, weight loss or body fat percentages. You don't need to down protein supplements (in fact, it could be best not to) or take gym mirror selfies. You don't even need a gym membership! Building fitness can be a gentle jog or brisk walk around the park, a Pilates class, weight training, boxing, interval training or doing your favourite team sport. Or it could be a dance class, aerobics or going on a hike.

The benefits of adding fitness into your world are huge, from boosting energy levels (and helping with quality sleep) to helping your cardiovascular and musculoskeletal systems thrive.[7] Your mood may also get a welcome boost from a heart rate-raising fitness session.[8]

Many people try to add fitness into the equation without the ground levels of the hierarchy of health being filled, which may result in a higher chance of injury, or make you less likely to keep up your fitness routine. Building up to fitness, so you can have a healthy, positive relationship with it, is pretty essential. Being well rested, hydrated and healthily fuelled will help you maintain fitness habits.

The thing to note is that your fitness and goals will constantly evolve depending on your life stage and specific needs. There is not just one way to do fitness; in fact, it's not a bad idea to try out different way to keep fit to keep things interesting.

How do you fare when it comes to fitness as a habit?

1. **How would you describe your level of fitness?**
    a. I'm not doing any or much exercise right now.
    b. I'd like to be fitter than I am.
    c. Good; I mostly have the energy to do things I want to do.
    d. Great; I am pretty dedicated when it comes to fitness.

2. **You want to get fit because . . .**
    a. I want to lose weight.
    b. I want to look a certain way.
    c. I mostly enjoy the process and know it is generally good for my mental and physical health.
    d. I love moving my body and feel like my mood, energy levels and mental and physical wellbeing are better for it.

Give yourself a point each time your answer was either an *a* or a *b*. If you scored 1 or more, then fitness is a habit that is yet to be acquired. If your experience has been tainted by diet culture, then working on fulfilling and enjoyable movement is a brilliant way to help shift your relationship with fitness, so it's not something you see as punishment for eating, but rather as a way to reward your body for existing.

How did you go?

You've now got a list of habits that might be missing from your life, in order of priority. In the next chapter, we're going to create a no-diet plan for helping you slowly and enjoyably fill in those 'habit gaps' and help you find strategies to make those changes. But first, there is one more level on the hierarchy of habits to cover.

Your ideal habits

Sitting on Level 4 are your ideal habits. This is the 'choose your own ending' part of the exercise. It's a chance for you to define and outline the habits you aspire to.

When you imagine your healthiest and most enjoyable life, what type of things would you do? When you've felt really good in the past, what habits did you find helpful? This could include habits like journalling, meditation, meal prep, growing vegetables or baking bread. These habits are the things you do when you're the dream version of yourself. It's your healthiest potential, for right now in your life.

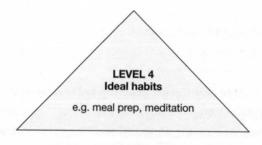

LEVEL 4
Ideal habits

e.g. meal prep, meditation

A Better Way To Be Healthy

These habits may help supercharge an already really healthy routine, which has been built up through working on the earlier levels of the hierarchy. In the next chapter, we're going to work together to build your ideal habits. I'll introduce you to three important questions that you can ask yourself to ensure these habits aren't accidental traps or a diet rule in disguise.

But before you do too much thinking about your ideal habits, please note that it's important that none of your chosen ideal habits be harmful to your body. The nutrition world has a history of willingly sacrificing one organ or aspect of health for supposed benefits; for example, advice to drink lemon water doesn't have any evidence to support the idea that it detoxes your body, but there is plenty of research showing how the acid can damage the enamel on your teeth, leading to cavities. Is it worth compromising the wellbeing of your teeth, which are critical for digestion, for supposed unsubstantiated benefits? Another example of this is unsupervised supplementation and herbal medicines, which, if unnecessary, can place an added burden on your liver and kidneys to process. This is the kind of thing I refer to as wellness wankery, and it's important to avoid it for the sake of your health.

Now that you know which blocks may be missing from your pyramid, it's time to start creating your unique, no-diet plan, starting from the bottom up, to help form healthy habits that stick.

Essential takeaways

* The hierarchy of healthy habits is a tool that can help you focus on the things that matter the most to your health.
* Filling in crucial 'habit gaps' in your hierarchy of healthy habits, in order of priority (starting at Level 1), is key.
* Many people skip important and essential core habits because of all the confusing nutrition messages.
* Creating a list of 'habit gaps' is a brilliant way to identify the most important things to work on when it comes to your health.
* There is no one-size-fits-all approach to health. Use the hierarchy as a framework to identify your health needs and gaps.

Chapter 5.

Create your no-diet plan

Health is different for all of us. That's all down to a little something called bio-individuality, which is just a fancy way of saying that even if you ate exactly what someone else ate and exercised in the same way, your body wouldn't look the same as theirs.

You're built differently (thank your biological parents for that), your hormones fire differently, plus your lifestyle is unique to you. As we've learned, what is healthy for you will change through different stages of your life. Just because you were once able to stick to a rigorous plan for months once upon a simpler (kid-free or stress-free) time, it doesn't mean that's where you're at right now.

That's why you're now going to customise your own no-diet plan to help plug the habit gaps you've identified in your hierarchy of healthy habits. Key to this is finding the right habits, and ensuring that they're actually doable. We'll take it step by step.

Step 1. Identify habit gaps

By this point, you've already completed step 1 by identifying your habit gaps back in Chapter 4.

Step 2. Test a new habit

Now it's time to begin the process of filling in those gaps, in order of priority. And this bit is important, because you'll want to ensure that you're not setting yourself up for failure by throwing any lofty, too-hard habits into the mix.

We often think we need to make huge overhauls in our lives to be healthier, but small, simple habits really do add up to something big. Research backs this up, confirming that taking on fewer habits, ideally one single habit at a time, is more likely to result in a behaviour change over the long term.[1] Instead of starting a hundred new habits on the first of January, adopt new habits gradually to give your brain, preferences and lifestyle time to change with you.

You're welcome to brainstorm your own strategies and habits. But here is a list of habits you might want to try on for size. They've been broken down based on elements within the hierarchy of healthy habits. Throughout this book, I'll be offering more strategies on how to address specific gaps in your hierarchy.

Un-sucky health habits to help fill gaps

LEVEL 1. BASIC NEEDS

Quality sleep

* Set a 'go to sleep' alarm so that your wind-down routine is completed earlier.
* Put your phone on charge in another room two hours before your bed time.
* Buy an alarm clock so you don't need to sleep with your phone next to your bed.
* Experiment with adding enjoyable movement to your day and see if it helps improve sleep quality.
* Speak to your doctor in case it's possible to identify other causes of your fatigue.

Eating enough

* Use your list of diet rules and work to unsubscribe from them, one by one.
* If you're ravenously hungry by mid-afternoon, it could be sign that you aren't having enough satisfying food that has long-lasting energy for lunch. Give yourself permission to eat until you feel comfortably satisfied. Try a salad sandwich, or a carb and protein-fuelled salad.
* If you're hungry, you probably need more than 100 calories or 12 almonds to feel satisfied. Check in with your hunger and allow yourself to eat until satisfaction.
* Try a pre-commute snack. Before you leave to go home, have a snack that truly fulfils your hunger, so by the time you arrive home, you won't be ravenous.

Hydration

* Have a glass of water (or more) with every main meal.
* Carry a water bottle that you enjoy using.
* Increase your intake of fruits and vegetables, as these are often loaded with water.
* Alternate alcoholic drinks with a glass of water.
* Aim for more alcohol-free days.
* A glass of milk will provide hydration, plus calcium and protein.

LEVEL 2. CORE HABITS
Managing stress

* Schedule time in your diary each week for self-care; for example, an hour each day or half a day on the weekend.
* Write a list of the things that feel stressful for you, identifying what is applying the most pressure. Tackle them one by one.
* Make an appointment with mental health–care professional (aka start going to 'gym for your brain').

Intuitive eating

* Before eating, check in with your hunger score (see page 148), asking 'Am I hungry?'
* Practise eating until you feel comfortably full, even if you're not perfect at it.
* Don't beat yourself up if you eat past fullness or eat before you're hungry. You don't have to do intuitive eating perfectly.
* When you eat past fullness, swap guilt for curiosity. When you eat more than feels comfortable, it's a chance to learn more about why it happened. Were you physically or emotionally hungry?

Cooking at home

* Stop making tasteless diet food. Embrace flavour and enjoyment. Try a new recipe each week to break free from a food rut.
* Cook at home one more night per week. Schedule it in your diary.
* When cooking, double the recipe so you have leftovers for lunch the next day (bonus: less takeaway will save more money).
* Ensure you have a sharp knife, a large chopping board and a frying pan as basic equipment.

* If you hate cooking, sign up to a cooking class so that you can get better at it (we tend to enjoy things we're good at). If you have the choice, an interactive class may be more useful than watching a cooking demonstration.

Enjoyable movement

* Find movement you genuinely like. Thinking back to what you enjoyed doing as a child can help you identify what would most excite you. Netball, dancing, swimming perhaps?
* Notice how your body feels when you go for a walk. Do you enjoy the process? Do you sleep better on the days you go for a walk or feel more optimistic?
* Ask yourself, 'How can I make movement feel more enjoyable?' Would music or a buddy help make it feel like a reward?
* Do you need different clothing so you don't chafe and jiggle? Get clothes that you feel comfortable in; nothing tight or itchy.

LEVEL 3. ENRICHMENT HABITS
Crowding and variety

* Try to include a different fruit or vegetable in your diet each week, allowing your grocery cart to shift with the seasons (and getting more diversity in your diet).
* If you usually eat the same kinds of vegetables, step outside your comfort zone and try something you haven't eaten in a while, perhaps prepared a different way. (e.g. Brussels sprouts cooked in an airfryer with a drizzle of balsamic glaze are delicious).
* Try new seeds and nuts or different spices and seasonings.
* Try a new cuisine type or one you haven't had in a while to mix things up. Try something you've never cooked or ordered before.

Mindful eating

* While you are eating, use your senses to appreciate the food. Enjoy the colours, smells, flavours and textures.
* Think about where the food came from and how it was prepared. Express gratitude for the meal and the people you share it with.
* Sit at the table to enjoy your meal. Avoid eating on the go or in front of the TV.

Fitness

* Set a goal that excites or interests you (run a 5k, do an ocean swim, complete a triathlon) and work towards it.
* Find a buddy that you can train with; this helps keep you accountable and is more fun.
* Get into a routine when it comes to training, working out at the same time each day so that it's part of your daily schedule.
* Make sure you fuel and hydrate your body appropriately, depending on the intensity of your exercise. If you're running long distances or exercising for extended periods, you'll need to replenish those energy stores.
* Find a good playlist or podcast to listen to while moving that wonderful body of yours.

Try my podcast No Wellness Wankery *for fun, diet-free advice on health, without the side serving of nutrition nonsense.*

Have you picked a habit that might help you fill in your habit gap? You may have selected a few that you could consider.

The three questions (for healthy habits that stick)

Before you consider shacking up with a new habit for good – or even for a weekend – it's got to prove itself by passing a test to help ensure your habit isn't accidentally a diet rule in disguise. If you can't tell whether you're doing it for the right reasons, refer to these questions.

Question 1. Does this bring me closer to the person I'd like to be?
Constructive habits move you towards the person you want to be. Neutral habits neither move you forward or hold you back, while destructive habits slow you down or move you further away from who you want to be. Does this habit help you get closer to your ideal version of yourself? If yes, then great! If no, then it's failed question one so it's not recommended right now.

Question 2. If this doesn't impact my weight, would I still choose do it?
This question helps rid yourself of habits you don't really enjoy, but you're willing to put up with if they lead to weight loss. It prevents you from getting trapped committing to something you don't really want to do, as it's unlikely to be a long-lasting habit anyhow. After all,

if doing a habit simply because it leads to weight loss worked as long-term motivation, wouldn't you be at your goal weight by now?

If there's a habit you enjoy doing that may also lead to weight loss, but you're doing it simply because you enjoy it or because you like the way it makes you feel, then it'll pass this test. But if weight loss is the primary motivator, then, sadly, it won't make the cut. Take running for example. If the only reason you want to run is to lose weight, you may not keep it up long term. If you do it because you enjoy it, whether it impacts your weight or not doesn't matter. It gets a green light.

Question 3. Can I maintain this for the rest of my life?

It might sound extreme but if you can't maintain this habit for the rest of your life, or at least for the next five or ten years, then what's the point in doing it in the short term? Even if you do get healthier temporarily, you'll likely slingshot right back to where you started as the health pendulum does its thang.

You might be willing to cut out carbohydrates for a few weeks or months – maybe even a year – but do you really want to spend the rest of your life trying to keep your body in ketosis or missing out on pasta?

You could do intense exercise that you don't actually enjoy to lose weight in the short term, but will you really want to still be doing this a year from now? Maybe you will. This question helps to figure that out.

Fasting intermittently may be fine temporarily, but what about forever? Dig deep and ask yourself honestly if it's right for you.

Wonderful Juliet tried going on a fasting diet without first asking the three questions. She shared with me, 'I feel like I have totally stuffed up my relationship with food in the last few years and I can't seem to find my way back. I think I really lost the plot when I started fasting with the 5:2 diet. I got this mindset of "the last supper" and going ballistic with food when I wasn't fasting. I ate every day like it was the last meal I was ever going to eat, because "tomorrow I will be good". I'm looking forward to letting all that go and just being able to eat like I used to.'

Asking yourself these three questions can help you easily decipher if something is dieting noise or if it's actually a sustainable habit for you. Because each of us is different and what feels restrictive to one person might be really enjoyable for another.

The three questions for making healthy habits that stick

1. Does this bring me closer to the person I'd like to be?
2. If this doesn't impact my weight, would I still choose do it?
3. Can I do this for the rest of my life?

Does your new habit pass these all-important questions? Did it get a green light? If so, fab. If not, cross it off the list and pick another habit to try on for size, running it through the checklist first.

You'll most often only ever stick to things that you enjoy. Ensuring your habit is actually enjoyable, so it never feels like a chore, is key. We'll talk about this more in detail in Chapter 8.

Step 3. Build on existing habits

Once a habit seems to be sticking around, even when life is stressful and chaotic, then it might be time to add another. Like climbing a ladder, take it step by step. Unlike diets with their massive pendulum swings, the aim is to gradually add additional habits. Patiently. One at a time, all the while listening to your body to see how it responds to each new habit (and by discarding any habits that no longer serve you). The end result is that you may look around a year from now, amazed by the steady progress you've made without depending on willpower, and without the volatility of those intense pendulum swings.

Once your chosen habit seems to be sticking around (for example, taking your dog for a daily walk) you can choose to build on it rather than adding an entirely new habit. You may gradually take longer walks, or go walking more often. One day you might find you naturally want to jog for a few moments while on this walk. At this point, you're successfully fulfilling your need for enjoyable movement and progressing towards finding fitness. After a year of progressively building up one habit, you might find yourself in awe of how you went from not walking at all to enjoyably running a few kilometres several times a week.

Another example? If you're trying to cook more at home, you might start by cooking one more night a week, progressively building up to cooking five times a week. You might then try to add more vegetables, aiming to get those five serves a day, practising crowding and variety. If getting to sleep earlier is your goal, but your current bed time is realistically midnight, aiming for a 9 pm bed time is probably too optimistic. You may start by trying to get to bed by 11:30 pm or 11 pm, gradually moving bedtime earlier until you've found your 'sweet spot'.

When to add another habit

Once a new habit feels easy and effortless, then it's time to add another new habit. It could happen after ten days or ten weeks. Some say it takes 21 days to form a new habit, while others believe it takes months.[2] Truth is, there is no magical formula or time period for how long a new habit takes to form. That all depends on the habit you choose, how easy it is to integrate the habit into your lifestyle and whether it's right for you right now. Once your habit is comfortably part of your homebase, that's when it's time to add in another one.

But when is a habit part of your homebase? If the habit is happening 75 per cent of the time, I consider that habit to be part of my homebase matrix. For example, I aim to go for a big walk every day. Realistically, though, I only get this done about five times a week at the moment. I don't feel guilty on the days I miss it, though I do crave movement if it's been two days without a big walk. But the point is, I still feel like I'm reaching my goal of moving my body most days.

Hooray for mental-health walks! Have you tried them? They're energising and stabilising.

Setting gentle goals

When setting your goals, it's important to allow plenty of flex room. Perfectly manicured and rigid goals don't work. Realistically, you don't need to execute a habit perfectly 100 per cent of the time to have reached your goal.

When you set goals, there is a tendency to set them as hard goals. For example:

* I want to love my body within a couple of months.
* I only want to eat when I'm hungry.

* I want to exercise five days a week.
* I don't want to overeat.
* I want to stop binge eating completely.
* I will stop talking badly about myself.

Keep in mind that 'eat when you're hungry' can easily be turned into a diet rule, so it's good to apply a gentler touch. Realistically, you won't always eat when you're hungry. Sometimes you'll have some lollies or chocolate fudge cookie-dough ice cream just because it's freakin' delicious. Saying 'I can only eat when hungry' is simply creating another dreaded diet rule. We've decided to give those a miss, yeah?

If you aim to eat when hungry most of the time, that's realistic and doable. It still leaves plenty of wriggle room for dessert or an almond croissant with a coffee. Also, 75 per cent of the time you may be able to accept or love your body, but there will still be days you doubt it. Because when you live in a world that is always telling you that you aren't thin or pretty enough, you won't always love your body.

There is something lovely about aiming to do something 'most of the time' while also allowing compassion for yourself when you aren't able to. What if you could consider a habit accomplished when it happens most of the time? Maybe you're already accomplishing more than you think.

Step 4. Experiment

Experimentation is the alternative to large overhauls in your life. It's an approach with listening to your body at the core of it. When you add a new habit, you're simply doing mini-experiments with your body. Not mad-scientist experiments, but simply testing a theory.

You might become curious:
* Will getting to sleep 30 minutes earlier help me feel better, be more relaxed around food or reduce out-of-control hunger?
* Does having oats for breakfast make me feel good for the rest of the day? Or do I feel better with eggs or avocado on toast?

* Is there a difference between eating dinner at the table versus in front of the TV?
* If I ate more for lunch, including carbohydrates, would it mean I'm less likely to raid the pantry and feel ravenous by mid-afternoon?

When you remove diet rules from your life, you're also running an experiment to test whether you feel better without that diet rule.

Experimentation is crucial when you adopt new habits. If it feels good, it's working. If it's feeling impossible, like a chore or it's rarely happening, then you take that as a nod from your body that it's not quite the right moment yet. It's not a reflection on your willpower or self-worth, it's simply a wink from your body saying 'not right now' or 'maybe later' or 'that habit was shithouse, let's try another one'.

Your body is constantly providing you with feedback; such as requesting more sleep or alerting you when it's ready for higher energy activities. From your bowels to your energy levels, your mood to how full you feel after a meal, all you're doing is becoming curious about how certain new habits make your body feel.

So when a habit doesn't work out, give yourself permission to ditch that habit, without an inkling of guilt. It could simply be time to try on another habit.

Perfectionism and procrastination

Are you a perfectionist? And maybe a bit of a procrastinator, too? These two are intrinsically linked. If you miss one workout, you've ruined your streak. Eat something you didn't intend to? That's the diet ruined, so eat whatever you want today and start dieting again tomorrow. Perfectionism tells us that if something isn't done perfectly, then it isn't worth doing.

Perfectionism ruins many things and health is just another casualty. If you're a bit messy or don't identify as a Type A personality, you might not immediately think of yourself as a perfectionist. But if you've ever thought, 'What's the point? I'll never get there!' or 'Today's already ruined so I'll start again tomorrow,' you might just be one.

Many of us try to chase perfect health. And why wouldn't we? Instafamous humans flaunt perfectly flat stomachs and their lives look pretty wonderful, traipsing around the Amalfi coast in bikinis. We think of health as avoiding all sugar, no alcohol, plant-based perfection with daily, rigorous exercise. The bar has been set too high. Chasing perfection turns you into a constipated turtle, unable to get moving or take action. You become crippled by anxiety and pressure, which is supremely unfun.

And it's not fun for the turtle either.

We give ourselves a hard time for not doing enough. Our self-talk stops us from making a start. Or when it comes to doing small things, you question if it's really even worth doing. You ask, 'What's the point of stretching my body if it doesn't burn enough calories? It's a waste of time' or we decide that, 'Yoga isn't real exercise because you don't sweat'. You dismiss activities that your body craves, that feel good to you, because they don't fit into the narrow, one-size-fits-all-approach that diet culture sells: that health is all about being thin, blemish-free and filtered.

When it comes to health, done really is better than perfect. It's likely that your 'perfect' vision of what it means to be healthy, as defined by inspirational day-on-a-plate videos or the countless diets you've tried over the years, is sabotaging your wellbeing. Much about health is simply turning up. Not aiming for perfect, but rather choosing to accept when 'healthy enough' truly is good enough. And then being able to enjoy the glorious consistency that comes from taking on less, making it doable and embracing imperfection.

In the English language, there is sadly no word that describes the magic of imperfection. Nothing to describe how 'perfect' can sometimes be a little boring and bland, predictable and lacking in character. And how sometimes the things we love the most are the unexpected, the mementos of a life lived deeply. Like my C-section scar from birthing my beautiful baby boy. Or the way someone you love snorts when they laugh deeply, and maybe farts too. Like when your biggest travel mishap somehow becomes the most memorable part of a holiday. The imperfect moments can be deeply touching; enchanting in their uniqueness.

There is a Japanese term, wabi-sabi – a concept often applied to design – which encapsulates this idea. Translated, it encompasses the appreciation for how imperfections can actually enhance the beauty of something, making it even better than if it was flawless.

When it comes to health, we could do with a little more wabi-sabi. Everything has become so curated, filtered, facetuned and done. We live in social media echo chambers, so often we end up replicating what we see others doing, instead of finding our own unique look, way of doing something or definition of health.

It's time to reject the too-hard-to-achieve perfect eating and the lofty exercise or body-fat percentage goals that make us feel like we're never quite good enough or doing enough. And lower the crushing pressure we feel to do it all, softening it to more manageable levels.

The end result: you're able to continue doing the things that make you feel good. You can take micro steps in the right direction because you're no longer fearful of getting it a bit wrong. You can finally break free from constant yo-yo dieting or obsession with clean eating and weight, and the accompanying self-loathing that comes with this nonsense.

What a relief it would be to lower the crippling expectations we have all been placed under, to reject this beautified and perfect-looking health ideal and choose ourselves instead. We would be healthier, happier and waste fewer precious shits on things that didn't matter.

Embracing imperfection looks like:
* removing the pressure you feel to do things perfectly
* choosing to take imperfect but consistent action towards your goals
* accepting that your body will always be bumpy and lumpy, and that it's not worth giving up your ideal life simply because you don't have your ideal body
* doing healthy things that feel good for your body even if it doesn't burn 'enough' calories
* caring more about how your body feels than how other people think it looks
* seeing a 'bad' photo of yourself and reminding yourself that it's not your job to look perfect from every angle (or ever!)

Imperfect consistency

Consistency. It's an elusive little beast. But it's the cornerstone of your health. You see, eating smoothie bowls and salads for a week isn't going to suddenly make you healthy in the same way that eating nothing but pizza for a week isn't going to destroy your health. It's only when you're consistently doing something that you start to yield an outcome.

In health, consistency is far more valuable than perfection. And in order to get more consistency, we need to lower our standards so that we can actually function and take care of ourselves. Going for a 20 minute walk every day (or even a five minute walk) is FAR better than aiming for an hour at the gym that never happens. Simply putting sunscreen on every morning is better than an elaborate skincare routine that only happens when Saturn crosses paths with Uranus.

Lowering your standards isn't giving up. It's quite the opposite. It's an outrageously smart thing to do. This simple act – doing easier things and expecting less of yourself – can actually help you get healthier without the pendulum swings or the paralysing procrastination.

What I'm saying is this. Imperfect action is better than no action. Done is better than perfect. And when it comes to your wellbeing, choosing to accept a little less in return for more consistency makes a lot of sense.

Of course, it would be great if you made your own yoghurt and meal prepped weekly, meditated daily and did all the things. And that's exactly what this book is about. Building small, healthy habits that feel doable, until one day they add up to something grand. The idea is that you might look around after having read this book and be tremendously impressed with just how much your lifestyle has changed. Or you might simply be finding that consistency is easier to come by, so even if there isn't a seismic shift in your habits, you're all the better for it.

Imperfection can help you:
* be more consistent
* feel better in your body
* make progressive steps to becoming healthier, building over time

* reduce procrastination (and improve self-esteem as you come to see yourself as the kind of person who gets things done)
* stop falling off the bandwagon or starting a new diet every Monday

My client Shona certainly feels this way, sharing that, 'It's so tough to find a balance between doing habits that make me feel good and making sure they don't feel punishing.'

Going on a diet is like putting up a tent for shelter. It's quick to get started, giving you an instant result. But you can't live in a tent for the rest of your life. On the other hand, building a healthier life is like building a home. Working through the hierarchy of healthy habits, you're making an investment in your wellbeing that takes time. You're taking the time to properly lay the right foundation, filling in gaps to ensure the structure of your health is sturdy, with a rock-solid base.

Ultimately, you don't 'get' healthy. You build health. Rather than going on a diet or turning to quick fixes, it's time to build real, long-lasting health.

You don't 'get' healthy. You build health.

Are you willing to be bad?

Some business advice I've received is that if you aren't embarrassed by the first version of a product you released, you waited too long to release it. The message? You have to start before you're perfect. Julia Cameron, author of The Artist's Way, says that in order to write a good book, you first need to be willing to write a bad book.[3] She explains that if you spend the whole time writing worrying if it's good enough, the perfectionism can cripple you, leading to writer's block. It results in empty pages. Nothing gets done. Which only whittles down your already sensitive ego.

It doesn't help when we now often see people doing things so effortlessly online, while we imagine that it must be effortless. And this world of quick online hacks tricks us into thinking it's all easy-peasy. So that when we try to apply it in our life and it doesn't feel as easy as they promised, we blame ourselves.

In an experiment conducted with toddlers, they presented the little ones with a task: to create a sound using a musical toy.[4] When the adult researcher presented the challenge as something 'simple and easy to do', the toddler gave up the task quite quickly. They assumed it was easy and so when it wasn't quickly achieved, they threw in the towel. But when the experimenter presented the task as something they would be challenged by, the toddlers persevered significantly longer. They understood the task was trickier. They didn't think the fault was intrinsic. They accepted the challenge, knowing they'd struggle a bit before it came good.

Health is not easy. It's not. It's hard to move your body some days. It's a lot to cook healthy meals for yourself all the time, to have written a grocery list and then made the time to cook it. While a recipe might be easy, many stars have to align for you to be able to have time to cook, have the ingredients on hand, the motivation to pull it together and juggle it all with what you feel like eating when you feel like eating. None of this is easy. Sadly, when we aren't able to do these supposedly simple tasks, oh boy, do we give ourselves a guilt trip over it.

In health, you don't need to do it well. You just need to turn up. And if you can't turn up, you have to give yourself grace and forgive yourself instead of believing you've 'ruined it'. Nothing is ruined. Expecting imperfection along your health journey is essential.

Softening your health goals is going to mean that it takes longer for you to arrive at your destination but if it results in more sustainability, more health and consistency, then it's the best option to take.

Are you willing to just show up with your health, and do it imperfectly? Start with the bare minimum? Begin with what's doable even though it might not feel extraordinary just yet? You have to trust that little things done often really do add up to something worthwhile. It's a real mindset shift.

Stop waiting

If I had waited until I was ready or good enough, I would have never started my business ten years ago and wouldn't be doing the work I love and have written a book. If I had waited to love my body to go to the beach, I'd have missed out on swimming in the ocean for 20 years. If I had waited to be brave enough to speak on a certain topic, I'd still be silent. If I had waited for the man who is now my husband to message me, we might not have met.

Stop waiting to get a flat stomach to wear a swimming costume. Stop waiting for your Instagram feed to make you feel better about yourself. Stop waiting to lose more weight to go on the date. Stop waiting for the world to tell you're good enough, or ready.

You don't need permission to start. If you wait to 'feel ready', you'll wait too long. Jump before you're ready, grow into the person you want to be. You've done enough waiting. The only way to finally feel like you're ready is by starting . . . and figuring it out along the way.

How to forgive yourself for not being perfect

It is not your job in life to be perfect or to get everything right. You do not need to look perfect from every angle or have everyone like you. Here's something I've learned. When you let go of the façade, stop trying to pretend you're perfect and reveal who you really are, it can be a relief, for yourself and also for others. When you turn up as you are, others can finally sigh in relief because they too now have permission let down their pretences and be who they are. It's a relief when we find out someone else also isn't perfect – just like us. And that's much more lovely than everyone pretending to be what they aren't. Don't ya think?

You have pores, occasionally a moustache when you haven't noticed it's grown back and tearful days when it all feels too hard. According to researchers in genetics, we all have on average about 60 mutations that occur in our bodies, given to us by our biological parents.[5] That could explain the weird birthmark or that hair that grows out of your left boob. I'm not suggesting you stop plucking that curly nipple hair (though you're welcome to if that lights you up!) or stop trying to excel at life, but I think it would help a great deal to be more accepting of our humanity.

Essential takeaways

* Once you've identified your habit gaps, it's time to pick habits to fill the holes.
* Choose one habit at a time, relating to the most important habit gaps you've identified.
* Using the three questions can help you make healthy habits that actually stick around and prevent you from getting trapped by dieting noise. The questions are:

   1. Does this bring me closer to the person I'd like to be?

   2. If this doesn't impact my weight, would I still choose do it?

   3. Can I maintain this for the rest of my life?

* Add a new habit, or build on an existing habit, when the current strategy starts to feel easy and effortless. If it feels too hard or is not happening as easily as you thought, then it's OK to ditch that habit and swap it for a new one, rather than staying stuck.
* Consider this process as an experiment. You're simply testing out a new habit to see if it works for you, checking in to see how it makes your body feel. Enjoyable and feeling good? Keep it. If it's too hard, it might not be the right habit for right now . . . or ever.
* Perfectionism is besties with procrastination. Expecting to be perfect can lead to paralysis and dread. It can lead you to try out habits that aren't right for you.
* Consistency is far more valuable than perfection. In order to get more consistency, we need to embrace the magic of imperfection.

Chapter 6.

Rebuild your energy

Quality sleep is a basic need and so is hydration.
Ensuring these basic needs are met are important steps
toward building up the hierarchy of healthy habits.
Ultimately, health isn't about having a cellulite-free
tush or a chiselled jaw, it's about having the energy
to do the things you love.

I recently caught up with my dear friend Gabi. A successful, kind and ambitious 32-year-old doctor who was struggling to meet her basic need of sleep. 'I've had a really tough couple of weeks,' she said, 'and today, I felt like I needed to cry. I knew it would make me feel better and I really wanted to cry but I just couldn't.'

'Why couldn't you cry?' I asked. She took a moment to think, paused, then said earnestly, 'Well, I was too tired to cry!' We both laughed because this felt so sad. And relatable. Not only was there no time to cry, but we're too tired to do it.

We are generation burnout. The social media–dependent, phone-addicted generation. Before mobile phones and emails existed, when you left the office for the day, you'd leave your work behind.

Leisure time wasn't filled up with feeds containing millions of potential pieces of content to consume. We spend hours on our smartphones each day, constantly glued to email or social media, with greater expectations around what can be done in just 24 hours.

Maybe we should refer to social media as 'addictive media', a more accurate name for the impact on our lives.

And it's seriously hard when you're taking care of tiny people. If you're a parent, weekends aren't really weekends. You might even look forward to Monday, or whatever day school or day care commences. It's not so much that we're craving the energy to chase after our kids so much as craving the energy to simply get through it all.

The worst bit about being an adult is that you have to parent yourself. Ever gotten to this point?

✷ I'm too tired to take care of myself.
✷ I put everyone else's needs above my own.
✷ I'm at everyone else's beck and call.
✷ It feels impossible to carve out even an hour of time for myself.

Burnout is affecting those with full-time jobs as well as stay-at-home parents, those whose workload never seems to end. This lack of real downtime, combined with the pressure we feel to match what we think other people are achieving, is bad for our health. It's impacting our sleep and our sense of self-worth. It's creating fatigue and malaise and disinterest. It means our lives stay small because we're so busy churning through the never-ending to-do list and never getting to enjoy true leisure time.

Society applauds us for working and being productive, even if it comes at the cost of our physical and mental health. Having a 'good work ethic' is seen to be a compliment, even if what it really means is someone who has sacrificed balance, their health or social life in order to work all the time. The things we can buy with the wealth we get from overworking are seen as social proof, something to be inspired by and revered, instead of people acknowledging the real life sacrifice being made.

We all consume so much productivity content – how to be more productive, how to get more done in a day, the routines of productive people, and so on – and it's no different to trying to squish our eating into the 'right' model or diet the way we 'should' for optimum results. If we switched to a more organic method of doing things we would be a lot healthier. If we trusted that we'd manage to fit it all in without constricting so much around it, I think we would all be happier!

Why am I exhausted all the time?

Reasons you might be excessively tired:
* lack of sleep
* energy mismanagement
* mental load
* diet burnout
* doomscrolling on social media
* iron deficiency

Yes, it could be low iron. Or another condition. If you are effing tired all the time, I do encourage you to go to the doctor for some blood tests to check if there is anything medical. This book isn't going to head into the potential medical causes for fatigue (of which there are many). Instead, I'm scratching the surface of the new phenomenon of burnout. Because many of us can relate to feeling like the world is asking too much of us and we don't have much more to give.

When I asked my social media followers, 'Do you feel tired all the time or burnt out?', about 82 per cent of people responded yes (out of 3,518 respondents). That's a huge number. And the constant busyness, striving, doing, hustle culture, perfectionism and pressure to fit into ideals has a tremendous impact on mental and physical health.

Our world has become so full and those everyday things keep piling up, requiring us to stay on top of them at all times. The result is constant overwhelm and fatigue, on top of the pressure to be the 'right' weight. Plus, there's the challenge of crappy sleep (not enough of it; poor-quality or interrupted sleep when it finally does happen) because you're too anxious about the bajillion tasks you have to complete each and every day to sleep easily. And even when you do manage to do all the things you're meant to be doing, why don't you ever feel satisfied?

And of course, there are days (or even periods of our life) when the pressure to do it all is too much and we end up doing nothing. This is followed by procrastination guilt, a very unfun and confidence-draining feeling that actually leads to MORE overwhelm.

What's more, emotional eating tends to happen when you have too many tabs open, or a seemingly insurmountable to-do list. In these cases, food can be used as a tool to soothe; a way to numb difficult emotions like overwhelm, mental fatigue, anxiety, sadness and more.

Energy management

Energy is the currency we exchange. It's arguably our most precious resource yet most of us are chronically depleted and tired. What's the point of having nice things that money can buy and free time if we're too annihilated to enjoy any of it? So we end up crashing on the couch on the weekends, trying to restore our energy just to get depleted again. Let's look at some key solutions to burnout, and for putting more energy in your body and mind.

Sort out your sleep

The problem is that we know we should go to sleep, but like a magpie, a whole bunch of shiny things are distracting and stopping us from getting to bed on time.

* ✶ 'Even though I'm exhausted in the afternoon, once I've done my priorities for the day, I'm too creative at night to sleep.'
* ✶ 'My brain is so active. I go to bed but then lie awake for hours.'
* ✶ 'I'm too busy looking after everyone else in my life.'
* ✶ 'The baby.'

There's a lot of chatter around how to get more sleep. I looked into a systematic review of literature that assessed the sleep patterns of more than 92,000 people.[1] Here are some of the key findings.

Going to bed late

Going to bed late is associated with depressive symptoms. People who go to sleep earlier and have more consistent sleep patterns are also reported to have a higher quality of life. If you're an early rising 'morning lark' opposed to a 'night owl' like me, you might go to bed earlier. As a result, morning larks tend to feel happier and more positive, potentially experiencing fewer mood disorders. Can you become a morning person? Yes, it seems you can. When you're younger, you might want to stay up later, but as you age, many people naturally start going to bed earlier and rising earlier too. This suggests that you might be able to switch from one chronotype to another.[2]

Social jetlag

Social jetlag is when your social life – or even your work life – is getting in the way of your natural circadian rhythm. You're having late nights, out socialising or working, even though your body would like to have a lie down. Social jetlag is when you go to sleep later and then wake up later on the weekends, then return to your usual sleep patterns during the week, creating a sense of jetlag, as though you're living between two time zones. The greater the mismatch between your time zones, the more social jetlag. And as with normal jetlag, social jetlag makes falling asleep harder. Social jetlag is often associated with sleep deprivation. This is why health advice is to try to have consistent bedtimes and wake-up times. It helps your body find its flow. And if you go to bed at the same time each night, you might find it easier to fall asleep and get enough rest.[3]

Set an alarm to go to sleep

A point I'd like to emphasise is this: instead of setting an alarm for waking up in the morning, try setting a 'go to sleep' alarm each night. This is your reminder to activate your wind-down routine. If you want to be asleep by 10 pm, this might mean a go-to-sleep alarm being set at 9 pm, allowing time for teeth brushing, face cleaning and hopping into bed and time to unwind with analogue enjoyment.

Weekend catch-up sleep

If you can catch up on some extra ZZZs on the weekend – or, well, anytime really, including a Monday afternoon snooze – this is a good move for your health. It's protective and may help to counteract not getting enough sleep previously in the week.[4] If you're a parent of little kids, this might mean napping when they nap. For parents with nap-free children, you could try tag-teaming with a partner on the weekend, alternating who wakes up early on Saturday or Sunday morning.

Essentially I'm saying that nothing is more important than your rest, especially not the laundry.

Sleep hygiene

Me telling you that you need more sleep isn't going to work. I've already mentioned the basics of 'good sleep hygiene'.

I recommend trying some or all of the following steps:
* Sleeping with your phone in a different room.
* Avoiding blue light, especially social media, close to bedtime.
* Not exercising close to bedtime.
* Sleeping in a dark room.
* Ensuring your bedding and room temperature are spot-on for the weather.

But it goes beyond good hygiene. Sleeping with my phone in a different room helps and all, but if I have kids waking up during the night or there are commitments I can't get out of or shift work, sleep hygiene isn't going to cut the wholegrain mustard.

Oversleeping

If you find you're always catching up on sleep, or sleeping ten hours a night, but you're still tired, it probably means your sleep isn't effective and this might be something to look into with your GP.

Consulting a sleep expert may be the support you need so the whole family can sleep better.

The key here is to recognise that you can't be your best self with poor sleep. Start asking yourself (or an expert), 'How can I improve my sleep?' Make it the priority that it should be.

Hydration

We forget to drink enough water: often it's not something we think about, or we don't like the taste of water (which can make things tricky). We turn our attention to other healthy habits, while neglecting this important component of health. It's part of the fuel that helps keep us moving. By making a few swaps, you can create a lasting hydration habit that you can build on further up the hierarchy.

What happens when you don't drink enough water?

Your brain is made up of about 73 per cent water. You probably already know that water does a whole bunch of essential things in your body.

It's important for:
* your digestive system
* avoiding or managing constipation
* producing saliva (essential for eating and breaking down food)
* making important hormones in your body
* cushioning your joints and supporting your bones
* regulating your temperature
* managing your blood volume, which impacts on blood pressure

A Better Way To Be Healthy

It's seriously not something you want to skip out on. Especially when you realise that being healthily hydrated is loaded with benefits. Getting enough H_2O into your body can improve sleep quality, cognition and your mood. It can impact your reaction time, memory and concentration levels.

That's not all. Your skin needs water, so it thrives and looks and feels better when it's well hydrated. Oh, and let's not forget about energy levels: when your muscles are dehydrated, they may fatigue sooner, which can leave you feeling flat. If I'm ever feeling tired, reaching for a glass of water has become a go-to to make sure thirst is not contributing to the fatigue. Ensuring that you drink enough water is a simple yet important way to help keep up your energy levels.

Realistically it could be the 138 emails I have waiting in my inbox, not lack of water.

Beyond aesthetics, your kidneys – the powerhouses that help clear your body of toxins – are grateful for the water you give them, allowing them to do their job well. Water helps your body break down food, and prevents constipation. Imagine the difference between trying to fling yourself down a normal slide while naked, or a water slide. Which would you pick? Water helps get things moving, and it feels a whole lot better too.

It's also worth noting that if you are thirsty but aren't drinking enough water, your body may try to access hydration in food form, meaning you end up eating when you aren't hungry. Ticking off the hydration box is therefore a good way to support yourself to be able to eat intuitively, trusting hunger to guide you based on your energy needs, not your water needs. But how much water do you really need?

Do I need to drink eight glasses of water a day?

Eight glasses of water is the general recommendation, based on the idea that we need to replenish around 1.2 litres (40 fl oz) of water each day. (We're constantly losing water through sweat, urine or by breathing it out.) But is the amount really the same for everyone? Not exactly. Someone who is 152 cm (five foot) doesn't need the same amount of water as a 192 cm (six foot three) person. A bunch of factors will determine how much water you use, including the weather, your muscle mass, activity level and what else you're eating or drinking.

Remember, alcohol comes in liquid form, but it's actually dehydrating.

How do you know if you're hydrated?

Thirst is a sign that your body is already dehydrated. Ideally, you should drink water before you notice thirst. If you are consistently thirsty, then you probably need to be more proactive with your fluid intake. Remember that your pee should be clear, light in colour or very pale yellow with a subtle smell. That said, some medications or supplements can alter the colour of your urine so it's brighter or darker. In which case, you'll need to use a different method to determine how quenched your body is.

Tip: If your wee isn't giving enough clues, constipation can also be a signal that it's time to drink more.

Some signs of dehydration include:

* feeling thirsty
* low energy
* dizziness
* feeling cranky or anxious
* headache
* muscle cramps

* constipation
* dry mouth or lips
* hangovers
* dark-coloured urine
* urinating less than four times a day

Note: feeling thirsty can also be a symptom of other things such as diabetes. It's a good idea to speak to your doctor and check that out.

How much water do you need?

* If you're running: Aim to have 150 ml (5 fl oz) of water for every 20 minutes of run time to help replenish the water lost as sweat. Endurance athletes would also need to add electrolytes.
* To help reduce the risk of a hangover: Aim for a ratio of 1 to 1, matching each alcoholic drink with a glass of water. Your body will thank you the next day.
* On a hot day: Sip on extra water. Smaller, frequent sips can be better than larger drinks spread further apart.

A Better Way To Be Healthy

Wellness or wankery? Weight-loss tea

The idea that any drink can make your liver, your body's natural detox machine, work overtime is crap. And that's also what weight-loss tea basically does, since they're usually caffeine, mixed with laxatives. Oh, and they'll dehydrate you while they're at it.

While they'll make vague claims about making you 'feel lighter', weight-loss teas aren't a magic solution. They're not going to boost your metabolism, burn away stomach fat, nor help you lose any long-term weight, other than water weight. Beyond that, they can be downright dangerous, since they're often unregulated, and abuse of laxatives has been linked to liver, gut and colon damage.

In other words, apart from messing with your bowels and brain, weight-loss teas are a pretty crappy strategy for any long-term weight loss. While we're on it, lemon water won't detox you either. But it will erode your tooth enamel, because of the citric acid in lemons. Ask your dentist. Skip fancy wellness drinks and choose water. It's very cheap.

Sadly, no one is going to remind you to sleep more, smell your wee to make sure you're hydrated or confirm you're eating enough. You've got to take care of you. And a beautiful place to start is by giving yourself permission to prioritise your basic human needs. 'Cause you'll likely be your best self with a little more sleep and water. Now let's make sure you're getting enough fuel.

Essential takeaways

* Quality sleep is a basic need and so is hydration.
* We are Generation Burnout. Instead of giving us more time to relax, social media and our devices eat up our freedom.
* Sort out your sleep with good sleep hygiene habits, which means your cat not your phone sleeps next to you
* Dehydration can affect more than just your health; it can affect your mood and your energy as well.

Chapter 7.

Heal your relationship with food

If you've used the hierarchy of healthy habits and identified that you may not be eating enough, or you think that your body may be confused about whether it's got a consistent and reliable supply of food, then this chapter is essential reading. It'll help you ensure you're meeting your basic need of 'eating enough food', without physical or emotional restrictions. But even if you feel this isn't an unmet gap, it may help to answer useful questions, like why you always feel like you have room for dessert or whether those cravings mean anything!

How to raid the pantry: a step-by-step guide

There's a sure-fire way to ensure you can't stop eating in the afternoon. This method also works for night-time pantry raids! Listen up.

Step 1. Don't eat enough satisfying food during the day. Spend the day 'trying to be good'. Opt for light, fluffy options, keeping a firm eye on calories. Keep snacks to measly portions. Stick to the recommended portion size or follow a meal plan and ignore your hunger.

Step 2. Arrive home ravenously hungry. Thanks to all the undereating you did all day, you're probably feeling outrageously hungry at this point. And there's likely to be a hefty side-helping of emotional hunger, too. As soon as you get home from school, work, university or the school pickup – or while enjoying your favourite TV show after dinner – you'll start eating and find it hard to stop! Well done. You have successfully dieted yourself into yet another pantry raid.

Step 3. Keep the cycle going. To ensure this happens on repeat, you're going to want to beat yourself up for it. Lather on the shame, guilt and blame. Promise to 'do better' tomorrow. This thinking will help you stay in this vicious cycle day after day. You might even find it gets worse over time!

Enough joshing around. I can't tell you how many people don't eat enough during the day. Or find themselves unable to stop eating after dinner thanks to emotional deprivation. How about we flip this cycle to work a lot better for us? It starts with understanding your body's starvation mode and the survival switch.

The survival switch

A few nights ago, I went to bed thinking, 'I don't want to cut out chocolate; I should just eat a bit less.' I'd just come home after a long weekend spent lounging on the couch, eating and drinking wine with good friends. And I'd accidentally taken on the guilt others were sharing about how they felt in their bodies.

The following morning, when I woke up, what was the very first thing I thought about? Chocolate. And I couldn't stop ruminating about just how much I wanted to eat it! It was playing on repeat in my mind. 'How can I get chocolate?' and 'is there any chocolate in the house?' It felt like quite an urgent need! An intense, desperate craving. What was that all about? Well, it seems I had accidentally triggered a primal, protective response. When your body fears that its supply of food is being threatened, it'll flick into survival mode; something I call the 'survival switch'. Luckily, because I noticed what was happening, I could take action to turn off my survival switch so I could go back to feeling normal around food again.

Later in this chapter, we'll dive into physical and emotional restriction.

What can flick on the survival switch?

* Physical restriction
* Emotional restriction
* Physical hunger

Simply planning to eat less is enough to make your body feel threatened. Telling yourself you must lose weight can do the exact same thing, even though you feel quite convinced deep in your heart that it would make you happier, healthier, more energetic. The survival switch is just one way your body protects you from real or perceived threats.

Any one of these things can flick on the survival switch:
* Thinking about going on a diet or trying to avoid a certain food (like I did with chocolate).
* Worrying about your weight.
* Stressing about what you ate that day.

* Allowing yourself to get too hungry.
* Undereating.
* Overexercising.

The survival switch is flicked on when your body fears there is a shortage of food. It can't tell you're dieting. It interprets a diet to mean that food is not plentiful. There's a limited supply. And your body does NOT like that. As a result, when you finally do get access to food, you may find you can't stop eating. That may be your body trying to protect you from the perceived threat.

Can you switch off the survival switch?

Yes. But your body has to feel safe again. Food trust is the knowledge that food is always allowed. That you can eat as much as your body needs, whenever your body needs it. Creating food trust is the essential step to help your body go back to feeling normal around food. The need to binge eat in secret may be reduced because you will learn that food isn't running out or restricted.

So when I recognised the early warning signs, here's the action I took to help my body feel relaxed around food again. I reminded myself, 'You don't have to avoid chocolate. You can eat as much as you need, anytime you want.' Phew. Within minutes of deciding this was true (not just muttering the words to myself while still holding on to hope that I could avoid the delicious options), I felt the energy change. I ate chocolate that day, but it wasn't a binge, just normal enjoyment of a food I loved. It could have turned out very differently if I hadn't noticed what was happening earlier.

This is a very handy saying to keep in your pocket:

I am always allowed to eat food. Nothing is off limits to me.

Best used as soon as you realise that you've flicked on the survival switch.

But here's the catch. You've really gotta mean it. No I'll-say-it-and-hope-it-works-while-secretly-still-trying-to-be-good nonsense. That'll backfire. You're welcome to try. I wish you luck! Send me a carrier pigeon if it is successful. But most likely, doubling down on your efforts to restrict may only make your cravings, bingeing or desire to eat stronger. You have to truly believe that any time you need more food, you are allowed to eat it. You can't say, 'Yes, but only if it's healthy' or 'only between these hours of the day' or 'only if it's dairy-free'. These things tend to make it worse.

The thought is this: 'If I want to have more of this food right now, I am allowed. If I want more in half an hour, in five hours, tomorrow morning or next week, I can always get more.' The way to flick off your survival switch is for your body to trust that food is always available to it. Your body needs to know that food is allowed, that there is no shortage or restriction on energy (food or drink). When your body stops feeling threatened, you'll switch off the survival switch.

For me, it took a few deep breaths and self-talk to switch off the survival switch. If your relationship with food is in a more turbulent place, it could take a while longer – days or weeks. It really depends on what your starting point is, whether you're actually willing to eat the foods you promised you would avoid. The problem is that most of us don't notice when this switch is flicked on. Instead, we blame our willpower. We think there's something wrong with us. The opposite is true. There's something very right with you. Your body is doing what it's designed to do: protect you, first and foremost.

TIP! Chronic dieters might notice their survival switch is very sensitive. It'll get flicked on with just one thought or tiny little trigger.

When it comes to triggering the survival switch, there are two big contributors that push you into the danger zone.

Physical restriction

Physical restriction is when you don't eat a certain food or you cut something from your diet. It's when you pass on the sweet stuff because you're trying to quit sugar. Eliminating specific foods due to IBS/IBD, reflux, intolerance or other reasons? This is also a form of 'physical restriction'. You're not meant to eat the food so you avoid it. And it can result in a similar experience to avoiding foods due to calories, fat or sugar. Like the participants in the Minnesota Starvation study (see page 28), you might become obsessed with the food you can't eat any more, even though you might need to avoid it for medical purposes or to feel good.

Portion control can be another form of physical restriction. If you're trying to cut down on the quantity of food by portion control, you might find you become obsessed with almost all food! People who tell me they binge or emotionally eat things like vegetables and fruit as well as chips or ice cream might be dealing with this problem. Your body might feel like it's being starved because you're physically limiting how much or what you're allowed to eat.

Note: If you're avoiding certain foods and it doesn't make you feel restricted, then that's not physical restriction.

Medical food restrictions: Trying to limit gluten but suddenly find you're binge eating it? Can't have dairy, but now you're eating a tub of ice cream more often than before you tried to cut it out? Applying food restrictions, even when they are necessary or important for you, can still lead to out-of-control eating. Most often the solution is to reintroduce the forbidden food and eliminate the guilt you feel when you eat it. You might find that you naturally choose not to eat this food when the choice no longer feels like a sentence.

Depending on the food issue, it's best to speak to an accredited practising dietitian.

Emotional restriction

Now, emotional restriction is a different, sneakier thing. It's when you tell yourself, 'I shouldn't be eating this food,' but you still eat it. You finish a meal and feel guilty about it, vowing that you'll avoid that food for a while. You exclaim to the group before dishing up, 'This is really naughty food' or 'I'm going to have to go to the gym tomorrow'. Or you try to limit how much of it you eat and then feel guilty when you eat more than you planned. You're still eating the food, and you feel bad about it when you do. This guilt and feeling like you've been 'bad' by deviating from your own diet rules creates a feeling of restriction.

Many frequent-flyer dieters are stuck in this confusing space of emotional restriction. After years of dieting, you might not necessarily be physically avoiding certain foods anymore but you're certainly emotionally restricting, beating yourself up when you do eat (hello diet burnout)!

Both forms of restriction – whether you're eating less or not – can make your body feel like you're not eating enough. It can lead to an obsession with food. And obsessing about food makes it very, very tricky indeed to just eat normally.

Now then. Do you think you're physically restricting or emotionally restricting (or both?) From my personal experience, many people (especially frequent dieters) do a mixture of both, alternating between the two at different points in their life. But almost everyone who has dieted is still emotionally restricting, leading to that intense, hard-to-pinpoint emotional hunger. Cue intense cravings; feeling crazy around food; struggling to just eat 'normally'.

Physical restriction *When you actually don't eat certain foods or physically limit how much you eat*	**Emotional restriction** *You tell yourself you're not allowed to eat certain foods (even if you still eat them)*
* Limiting portion sizes. * Weighing out food. * Counting calories, macros or points. * Avoiding foods you think are 'fattening' or 'bad'. * Avoiding foods because of a specific diet, such as IBS, coeliac disease or reflux. * Cutting out whole food groups, such as sugar or carbs. * Time-based eating, such as intermittent fasting. * Not allowing yourself to eat after a certain time at night. * Feeling hungry after eating because you didn't eat enough.	* Telling yourself you're only allowed to eat a certain portion size regardless of your hunger levels. * Feeling guilty for eating certain foods . . . or any food! * Worrying that others will be judging you for eating certain foods. * Having a list of 'bad' or 'red' foods you aim to avoid. * Food rules.

A Better Way To Be Healthy

✎ What triggers your survival switch?

Becoming aware of what triggers your survival switch (see page 124) and noticing when it happens can be seriously helpful stuff. It may help you avoid slipping into I'm-feeling-crazy-around-food mode before it even happens or help you recover from it faster. Answer the following questions:

✸ **Was I physically hungry?** Not sure? The hunger scale (see page 148) will be able to help with answering this question.

✸ **Was I emotionally hungry?** Did I feel deprived? Was I accidentally subscribing to a diet rule?

✸ **What triggered me to feel out of control around food?** Write down the exact incident that happened and the thoughts that followed.

You can decide not to subscribe to the thinking that comes from the trigger. You may enlist some new thinking to help counteract the old ideas, challenging the idea that the thoughts you had in response to the trigger are 'fact' and helping to shift the way you bypass the survival switch.

✎ Identify your triggers

Here's an example.
Incident: My mother-in-law commented on how much weight my sister-in-law has recently lost.
Feelings: It made me feel that I should lose weight. I felt judged and maybe jealous, too.
Thoughts: I need to lose weight. I'd be better off and get more praise.
New thought: My mother-in-law's comments are a reflection on her relationship with her body, not my body. I'll keep focusing on my health.

Here is another example.
Incident: I was out for lunch with a friend. After eating half her meal, she said she was full and stopped eating. I wasn't nearly full!
Feelings: I felt worried that there was something wrong with my appetite, and guilty for needing more food than her.
Thoughts: I should stop eating now even though I don't feel full. Maybe she thinks I'm a pig for eating the whole thing. Maybe I always overeat.
New thought: I am allowed to eat as much food as my body needs. My appetite is perfectly attuned for my body.
Find a free worksheet on my website, *lyndicohen.com/bookresources*.

Are you addicted to food?

Or are you simply not eating enough? Do you ever feel crazy and out-of-control with food like you just can't stop? Shereen was convinced that she was addicted to sugar. After all, what else could explain her need to have something sweet after every meal or her obsession with cookies-and-cream ice cream? 'For many years I have believed that I am addicted to sugar. They say sugar is eight times more addictive than cocaine. Do you think this is true? Can we be addicted to sugar? I know once I start eating something sweet my control leaves me.'

She signed up to an abstinence group, trying to do what she thought was right to fix her 'sugar addiction'. In Shereen's own words, 'No matter how hard I tried, I could never attain total abstinence of sugar and "white" foods for more than a day and was constantly besieged by bingeing and cravings.'

There is much debate about this question. Some people argue you can be addicted to food, but I do not believe it. And there are researchers who would agree with me.[1] You see, unlike alcohol or cigarettes, your body NEEDS food, including things like sugar (carbohydrates) and other components of food such as fat or sodium. Your brain and muscles require glucose and glycogen to function (these are forms of sugar). Is it really fair to say you're addicted to something you require to stay alive? It's like saying we're addicted to water or air. Food is not an addiction. It's an essential ingredient to human survival.

If you feel addicted to food, then the real problem may be your relationship with food, including things like sugar. All that restriction from dieting has led to these food obsessions. So like a toddler told they can't have or shouldn't do something, it only makes it more appealing. Telling yourself you're addicted to sugar and that it's terrible for you may only increase the primal desire for the very thing you NEED to survive – food.

Nutrients aren't everything

It matters how satisfying you find a certain food. I mean, it really matters a lot. People often beg me to tell them which are the healthiest foods. Berries or kale? Surely you need to limit sugar and fat, right?

We think good nutrition is about getting the right mix of nutrients and avoiding the wrong type. You've been taught to count grams of sugar to tell if a breakfast cereal is healthy or limit grams of fat. But just looking at the nutrients without considering how fulfilling the food is can make it hard to stick to healthy eating. Because while kale might be healthy food, humans choose foods that are satisfying. Taste and fullness are more important to our primal need for fuel than micronutrients.

One of my clients, Jo, shared their take on it: 'I was so focused on only "clean" and healthy eating that I was missing the aspect of moderation and enjoyment. I was eating only plain, high-protein (low calorie) yoghurt as a snack and never really found it satisfying. I'd find myself then raiding the cupboard half an hour later and eating lots of sweets or other foods because it never really satisfied me. Now I just have either a flavoured yoghurt or a plain yoghurt with a spoon of honey or jam and it satisfies me so that I don't actually go back to binge. This is so liberating, because not only do I enjoy my snack more (even though there are more calories in it), I also am not fixated on food afterwards and don't binge because of this! It has made me feel so, so much better and has helped me to stop wasting time thinking about food and actually have time to do things which I enjoy.'

Satisfaction REALLY matters

How do you know which foods are more satisfying than others? Well, tuning into your lovely body after you eat certain foods is going to be a fantastic guide. Diets have taught you to tune out of bodily sensations in place of 'good or bad' thinking.

The 1995 Satiety Index of Common Foods offered an insight into which foods were actually more satisfying to eat. And the results are quite interesting.[2] The most satisfying food, according to the study, was boiled potatoes, a food which has been banished from the health world for many years. But anyone who's eaten boiled potatoes can confirm this is a deeply satisfying food. When you finish a meal with boiled potatoes you're likely left feeling like you've actually eaten, unlike after you've finished a nutritious (but unfulfilling) smoothie.

According to the Index, other foods that are very satisfying include porridge, white fish, red meat, grainy bread, brown pasta, beans and sauce, apples, oranges, grapes, rye bread and bran cereal.

What I find most interesting about this list is that many of these foods are on the banned or forbidden list in many diets. Potatoes, porridge, bread, pasta, beans and fruit aren't included in popular low-carb diets, while cutting out fish and red meat has become a trend as part of the plant-based movement. Some of the most satisfying foods are the ones that have been demonised and we've been told to cut out, limit and avoid.

Do you know what happened? By avoiding these satisfying foods, we are making it harder to end our meals feeling truly satisfied. If you build a diet on nutrients alone, without considering how satisfying a meal will be, you end up creating a diet that is near impossible to stick to.

Fruit is another food group that we've been taught to fear thanks to the sugar-phobia of late. Yet, this index found that higher-sugar fruits can actually help you feel more satisfied (compared with high-fat foods). This makes sense. While berries are touted as antioxidant rich and low in sugar, I don't find them very satisfying. Plus, when I'm truly hungry, I'm not really tempted to reach for the berries because I don't think they're going to hit the sides of my stomach. When I have done this in the past, the berries become my appetiser and I invariably end up searching the pantry or fridge for something to take my hunger away.

Personally, I can demolish a punnet that cost me $5, without even feeling like I've eaten.

This is quite different from eating a banana or mango. Not only am I happy to reach for one of these (yum), but they shift my hunger, leave me feeling satisfied so I'm less likely to keep rummaging for more food. My brain is free to get back to living my life. Yes, these fruits do have more sugar and energy. Demonising perfectly healthy foods like fruit can be self-sabotaging.

Snake meal

What is a snake meal? It's when you don't eat for the entire day then consume a million calories in one meal, like a snake. It isn't an official medical term, but it should be!

Some cleverer alternatives to a snake meal:
* Noticing your hunger and responding to your hunger.

A Better Way To Be Healthy

* Having a pre-commute snack.
* Preparing lunch for yourself at the same time you prepare food for other people (you know, fit your own mask first . . . or at least simultaneously).
* Scheduling a lunch break. Speaking to your boss to ensure you have eating breaks while at work or school.

> **SNAKE-MEAL TIP!** Avoid the temptation to skip breakfast the morning after a snake-meal feast. You may be tempted to try and undo what you ate during the snake meal. This will likely lead to another snake meal. Don't do it. Be smart, you silly reptile.

More satisfying food

Which foods are more satisfying for you? Are there foods you currently avoid that are actually really satisfying for your body?

Some common satisfying foods my clients have been taught to avoid:

* Pasta
* Rice
* Bread
* Fruit
* Wholegrain cereals
* Beans and legumes
* Starchy vegetables like corn, potatoes

We've got to break from thinking that you can't eat pasta or bread to be healthy and swap it with the understanding that these foods play an essential (and deliciously satisfying) role in a sustainable diet. What would happen if you allowed more satisfying foods into your diet?

At 46 years old, Margaret shared her moment of liberation with me. 'I was hopeful but a little sceptical that I'd be able to break down 20 years of dieting behaviours and beliefs, but yesterday was something of a turning point. At home with little in the fridge and no time between meetings to get out and shop, I hunted around for lunch at about 2 pm when I was actually hungry. I had none of my "good" foods left, so typically I would have resorted to skipping a meal, snacking on chips and biscuits meant for my daughter's lunchbox, and then overeating at dinner. Instead I let myself have two slices of sourdough loaded with fresh tomato and a sprinkle of salt and pepper. It was so delicious and I can't believe I've missed out on eating foods like this because "bread is bad". This is going to be a game changer for me: I already feel less anxious about my next trip to the supermarket.'

You can include these foods in your diet if they make you feel good. This might mean instead of avoiding carbs, you include pasta as part of your diet or use brown rice as the base for a meal. Make a tray of roasted vegetables including potatoes along with other vegetables. Or have a potato-rich meal, enjoy it and then move on with your life, revelling in the satisfaction of eating something that allows you to stop thinking about food until you next get hungry. If 'perfect' eating is about only having 'allowed' low-carb vegetables, 'healthy enough' eating embraces a lovely mix.

The need to finish everything on your plate

Maybe you can relate to Jenny and her experiences? 'I grew up with a loving family who loves to eat. This caused me to feel "obligated" to finish my whole meal when it's on my plate, even if I'm full! I was raised with Mum dishing up my dinner and I had to sit at the table and finish everything or it would be served to me cold for breakfast. I don't think I've got a well-developed sense of when to stop eating. Also I have 40 years of programming telling me it's wasteful and wrong to throw any food away and I must finish what's on my plate. When my daughter was little I even used to finish up what she didn't eat rather than throw it away.'

If you can relate to Jenny, there are a couple of phrases worth trying next time you find you're already full but eating just to make sure the food is finished.

Phrase 1: 'Food is wasted if it ends up in the bin, but it's also wasted if it ends up in my body and I wasn't hungry for it.' It's simply a different kind of waste. Whether in your body or the bin, it's still wasted.

Another thing to consider is how, when we are dieters, we have a niggly sense of emotional restriction that's always lurking. Our brains tell us we really shouldn't be eating this or we have an underlying belief that food may run out at any given time (especially potent if you

✎ What to do after you eat more than planned

Here's a user-friendly summary for my snake-meal friends.

1. Push back against guilt. Resist the temptation to beat yourself up for eating. Remind yourself of these important things:
    - ✻ I'm always allowed to eat to satisfy my hunger. If I'm hungry, my body needs more energy and I should eat to feel satisfied.
    - ✻ I do not need to eat perfectly in order to be healthy.

2. Return to your homebase. The day after you found you couldn't stop eating, fight the temptation to diet or undereat, to swing that pendulum wide. The aim is to return to your homebase of habits. Start the day by tuning into your hunger. If hungry, try a decent but normal-for-you breakfast. Then wait to feel hungry again.

3. Make sure you're eating enough during the day. Here's one thing (of many) I know to be true: If you undereat at one meal, chances are you'll end up eating more at the next meal. The problem with undereating at breakfast or lunch (there's that pesky 'trying to be good' fallacy again) is that you're more likely to overeat or binge because you're burnt out and starving from running on empty.

4. Ensure your food is satisfying. If you find you don't feel satisfied after a meal, you probably need to eat more. You're better off eating a substantial lunch full of healthy fats, slow-burning carbs and lean protein, a powerhouse trio that'll keep you energised while you're running around being your best self. A solid lunch may mean you can happily enjoy a lighter (albeit balanced) dinner before lying horizontally for, ideally, 7+ hours.

grew up without a steady source of food). Feeling the need to finish everything on your plate – and other people's food – can be caused by food scarcity, a result of dieting.

Phrase 2: 'I am allowed to eat as much as I need to feel satisfied. If I want more of this food later, I can eat it.' As I've mentioned already with this phrase, you've really got to mean it when you tell yourself it. You can't turn it into another food rule, something to try to curb eating. You've got to really help your body trust that this food or other food is truly always available.

Knowing that food isn't going to run out, that there is enough (or more than enough) and listening to your body when those cravings strike are key parts of creating a healthier relationship with food. And an important essential need to fulfil in your hierarchy of healthy habits.

Normalising forbidden foods

Do you eat perfectly in front of others but binge eat in secret? If so, it's time to normalise forbidden foods. How? Well, instead of waiting to eat these foods when no one is looking (for fear of judgement), you choose to eat them in more public and social settings, with full permission. If you binge on chocolate, you might order choc-hazelnut spread on wholegrain toast at a cafe. Is the spread healthy? No. But if it saves you from bingeing later, then you're much better off. You still have other meals in the day where you can practise crowding in more healthy stuff so that over the course of the day, you don't eat perfectly but you avoid a binge and still include plenty of healthy options.

Another example? You might go for a sweetened yoghurt when you feel like something sweet. Is it better to have plain Greek-style yoghurt? Of course. But if having a little bit of sugar in your yoghurt means you avoid a binge later (which could mean much more sugar), then it's worth it. What I'm saying is: stop trying to eat perfectly. Start trying to eat 'healthy enough'. It's much gentler, and much more doable.

Controlling food to control life

Life is chaotic, hard and messy. Often, trying to control food isn't just about weight or how you look. It can also be an attempt to control something in a very uncontrollable life. It's a bit like how you might find it hard to relax when your house is a mess.

If your immediate environment is neat and orderly, your brain can be tricked into thinking that life is more under control. The same applies to food. If your eating is 'in order' or under control, then it can help make the rest of your life seem more managed. This may also explain how, when you feel out of control around food, it can lead to catastrophising and a feeling like everything is out of place. It's the pressure to get on top of this weight thing. This is yet another reason why the need to diet and control food feels so compelling that we prioritise it and allow it to take over.

We have this idea that the more we control food, the more control we will have over food. But the opposite often happens. Gloria experienced this first hand: 'Right now I keep eating emotionally and am scared I will keep gaining. I eat a healthy balanced diet and enjoy cooking healthy foods. But because of my emotional eating, I'm finding it hard to feel like I'm in control. A healthy, balanced relationship with food would have me not obsessing over food, not overeating and fuelling my body with what it needs to feel its best.'

In a very real way, believing your weight is the problem provides a relatively clear focus. It distracts you from all the real challenges of life, the loss, the parents with too many expectations or the disinterested parents. It's a distraction from the things you can't get right, the hardship of growing up, of being left out, the grey of life when what you really crave is clarity: black and white is easier to live by.

And diets give us black and white. They give rules to follow based on equations: 'This is SCIENCE! You can trust us,' diets scream in shiny marketing. All you have to do is follow these instructions, this meal plan and be a good girl. Dieting provides a very welcome distraction from tricky things in life. It starts off being fun. Oh, how I always loved the motivation and enjoyment you get when you start a new diet, you're in the zone and the compliments start flying in. You feel on top of the world. And this state propels you forward, keeping you focused. (Until that is, the health kick wears off or you diet so often that you don't even get this feeling anymore due to diet burnout).

Emotional and binge eating

Almost everyone does some degree of emotional eating. Research explains how feeling emotional or bored can lead us to experience cravings.[3] But I guess we probably didn't need research to tell us that. We're emotional creatures!

I'm still glad they did the study!

But dieting can really supercharge emotional eating. We eat for three main reasons: hunger, enjoyment or coping. Like taking drugs, drinking alcohol or overexercising, eating food is a coping strategy. What happens when you stop allowing yourself to eat for enjoyment –

by placing diet rules and bans on food – is that you may depend more on food for coping. Food becomes more powerful at soothing you (albeit temporarily) when you remove food as an item for enjoyment.

Mindful emotional eating

You don't need to try to eliminate all emotional eating. Some degree of it is normal. So often, we are emotionally eating and don't even realise we're doing it. But you can start to try to recognise when it's happening, without judgement. For example, you might say to yourself, 'I've had a hard day. I am emotionally eating right now to make myself feel better.' Already, simply becoming mindful when it's happening is a huge step.

When you emotionally eat and then you add guilt, followed by restriction, that's when something quite normal can spiral into binge eating. Like Jess, who said, 'I know EXACTLY what I should be doing but I can't seem to get back in that mindset. Even now, I eat something terrible and I know how many calories are in it and the shame and guilt makes me binge more.'

Binge eating

Binge eating can feel quite different from emotional eating. It's when you feel out of control around food. While you're having one mouthful, you're probably already planning your next. You feel like you can't stop. And you may eat way more than you normally would. Plus, binge eating might be something you find you do in secret. With emotional eating, you may or may not do it with friends or in front of family as it isn't as tied up with guilt and shame. That's why with binge eating, you might try to hide empty wrappers. You might notice you feel guilty, ashamed or angry about how much you ate.

These feelings of shame and guilt can lead you to restrict your food following a binge, which only serves to further boost physical and emotional hunger. As a result, another binge is almost inevitable.

Katie's story explains this vicious cycle quite well: 'I recently lost weight by restricting all of the foods I loved: this included cereals, pasta, breads and snacks. However, since then I have been severely bingeing. Pretty much every single day. I will hide in the pantry and binge. It's almost always on bread and cereals. I could eat five wraps in one go. I cannot stop until I am sick to the stomach. And then of course following this binge is the regret, guilt and the obvious weight gain over the last few months due to the bingeing.'

Binge eating is something that – if you don't get treatment for it – can get progressively more frequent and more intense. Like with my experience. Every time I tried to double down on my weight-loss efforts after a binge, the more out-of-control my binges became, until I was eventually binge eating multiple times a day.

When to get professional help

Overeating occasionally is one thing but when you start to feel out of control around food, find you're eating way more in a sitting than you normally would, feel guilty about it . . . and find it's happening pretty often, it may be time to get professional help. Make an appointment with your GP and explain your binge habits to them. You may be referred to a specialist dietitian who can support you on your journey. And of course, there is always my Keep It Real program. Visit *lyndicohen.com/keep-it-real*.

Cravings

Does this ever happen to you? You try to have a 'healthy' snack, which is code for a low-calorie, 'good' snack that is allowed based on your personal set of diet rules, but what you really feel like is some chocolate. Or salty chips. But you push that feeling to the side and you reach for your healthy alternative to try to sidestep the cravings. You grab a handful of nuts instead. Hmm, still not satisfied. Maybe some yoghurt will do the trick? You eat it. Still no dice. Some biscuits then? You then proceed to eat 293 other things, that progressively get less and less healthy, before eventually eating the chocolate or chips anyway. Then you feel like a failure.

Read any health publication or news site and it'll probably take you 0.23 seconds to stumble upon some article claiming to help you 'resist snack temptations' or 'curb your sugar cravings'. It's a thing.

The irony is that the clichèd advice – to avoid the craving – may be leading to this avalanche of eating. It's causing emotional hunger, coupled with guilt, making it hard for you to actually enjoy the thing you wanted to eat in the first place. People who have dieted are more likely to experience cravings. And we've talked about how avoiding food is probably going to cause a spike in cravings for the forbidden food. This is why trying to banish cravings may have the opposite effect, leading you to a stronger desire for the very food you're trying to avoid. Dang. Just another example of how the advice you've been dished out by diet culture has made healthy eating harder.

What these health articles neglect to tell you is that the best way to cure a craving is to eat the thing you're craving. Eat it mindfully, with full enjoyment (not with a side serving of guilt), and then move on with your life.

Does this mean you should just eat junk food all the time and neglect your health? No. That's not what I'm suggesting. You can still aim to crowd in lots of healthy options, filling your house with nutritious, easy-to-grab choices, but when those cravings inevitably do strike, you can easily respond calmly and with enjoyment, without it cascading into a blow-out, a bigger thing than it needs to be. This is very much the strategy those 'normal' non-dieters seem to adopt. And they tend to get fewer cravings than we dieters. Can you see how avoidance makes the problem worse, leading to more cravings and more intense cravings?

Craving myths

There's a myth that cravings are a sign that your body doesn't have enough of a certain nutrient.[4] The idea is that if you crave chocolate, you're deficient in magnesium. Craving bread or pasta? Then you're supposedly low in calcium. Oh, how I wish this were true; what a simple world that would be! You could simply take supplements to fix chocolate cravings and it would – poof! – disappear. Sadly, cravings don't mean you're deficient in a nutrient.

This is just another example of a health myth that gets perpetuated by the media.

That's not to discount cravings, which are a seriously real phenomenon – just ask almost any woman and she can confirm. There are gender differences when it comes to cravings. Ninety-seven per cent of women compared to 68 per cent of men experience cravings.[5] Ha! Hormonal hunger and dieting history may help explain this.

Turns out, the most commonly craved food is kale. Just joking. It's chocolate.[6] Obviously. Chocolate takes the prize and by a long mile. In general, craving something sweet is more common than craving savoury food, especially among women.[7]

This is true in Western countries, but in Egypt participants were more likely to crave savoury food!

A new relationship with cravings

When you first quit dieting, there will be a period when you still have lots of cravings. Suddenly allowing yourself to eat the foods you've been avoiding for years can do that. But with time, as you continue to remind yourself and teach your body that it really can eat chocolate or chips – it's a choice, not a law – then those cravings can start to reduce in frequency and intensity.

Essential takeaways

* You're probably not addicted to food. Depriving yourself of your favourite foods can increase cravings.
* Giving yourself permission to eat these foods, 'normalising' them, may help you feel more relaxed around food in general.
* The survival switch can get flipped on by dieting, or even just thinking about going on a diet. This is a protective mechanism.
* To turn off the survival switch, you need to help your body know and trust that food is plentiful and always allowed.
* If you do eat more than you plan to, instead of dieting, follow the steps outlined on page 135.
* You can eat as much as you need to feel full. Choosing satisfying foods will help. Reminding yourself that you can always have more when you want to eat again can help (but you really have to mean it)!
* Cravings are common and normal.

Chapter 8.

How to eat intuitively

Oh, it's getting juicy now! We're about to talk about core habits, which sit on the Level 2 of the hierarchy of healthy habits. While not essential for basic survival like Level 1 habits, don't be deceived. Core habits can help to make your life luminous and your health better. And a seriously important habit within this mix is intuitive eating, which is the act of tuning in to your wonderful body's innate hunger and fullness cues.

We all know there is a big difference between fashion and personal style. Fashion is about keeping up with the trends; following what everyone else is doing and constantly trying to keep up. It is short term, a huge contributor to landfill and will probably make you scratch your head in 20 years' time when you stumble upon a photo of yourself with a permed mullet.

On the other hand, personal style is about cultivating your unique approach to dressing yourself. It's the art of listening to what makes you feel most like yourself, the most brilliant and energised version, and then refining that style over time. It's a process of experimentation, of listening to what works and throwing out what didn't work. It's a long-term pursuit that results in a timeless look that is true to your essence.

Chasing diets is like chasing fashion trends. You need to cultivate real health the same way you cultivate your style.

If you only take one thing from this entire book, please make it this. You are the expert on your body. As long as the diet industry continues to profit off our insecurities, shouty magazines and so-called experts will continue to promote the latest diet trend. There will ALWAYS be a new diet or thing to try. What if, instead of chasing shiny new trends, you invest in understanding what works for your body, what is timeless for you?

Your body is constantly trying to communicate with you to help you take good care of it. If a food makes you feel bloated and yucky, even if it makes other people feel great, it might not be the right food for you right now. If exercising in a certain way – like going for walks – makes you feel great, then it's a good choice for your body, even if you've been told high intensity interval training is the 'best' thing to do.

Learning to listen to your body is one of the most important things you can do for your health. And key to this is becoming aware of hunger and fullness.

Physical hunger

Physical hunger is perhaps the most obvious form of hunger, so let's start here. If you've ever been told to 'finish everything on your plate' or tried to stick to a meal plan with regimented 'ideal eating windows' or portion-size guidance, this is going to be a revolutionary concept.

Human instinct is a wonderfully clever thing. You instinctively know when you're tired or when you need the bathroom. You don't need to consult a special health book for optimal bathroom breaks. Since kindergarten, you've taken cues from your body and (mostly) avoided peeing your pants on purpose. Wonderful work. Gold star! When it comes to hunger and how your body signals how much to eat, it's down to another instinctive mechanism: your appetite. And if you can tune into it, it can help to regulate your body's real-time needs. No diet subscriptions necessary.

Key to this is trust. This is where intuitive eating comes in. Your body is constantly communicating with you about how to best look after it. And by learning to respond to your body's needs, you may be guided to make food choices that feel good, without judgement.

How appetite works

Your appetite is essentially a very clever, built-in weight and energy management system. A way for you to know how much sustenance your body needs at any given time, specific to how much energy you're using. Your appetite is a nifty and much-underrated tool to help you eat for your body's needs.

Your brain and stomach are in constant communication with one another. A super-smart section of your brain (the hypothalamus) receives chemical messages from your gut and fat cells letting it know that you're hungry. Your body translates these messages and determines that it is time for food. 'More energy, please!' your cells request. Hunger is your body's way of letting you know how much or how little energy to take in.

Before you were asked, 'Do you really need to eat that?' or someone suggested you don't need second helpings, you were a child. You'd peer into the pantry, wondering what to eat based on your hunger, what was tasty and how it'd make you feel. You didn't do mental arithmetic before deciding what to eat and you certainly didn't spend much time mulling over whether what you ate that day was right or wrong.

As a kid, you probably ate intuitively, letting your hunger and energy levels guide your food intake. You didn't finish the packet because 'the diet starts again tomorrow'. And because you knew you could always have more food if you wanted, you didn't feel the need to eat to discomfort. Such simple times.

Generally, children have a pretty carefree relationship with food. They are healthy, intuitive eaters. That's because they're yet to be indoctrinated into diet land, a world where food rules and exercise expectations dictate what, when and how much we eat.

Perhaps you have noticed that some days you are ravenously hungry? On these days, your body may be using more energy. On days when you are less hungry (and may even forget about food), your body is potentially burning less fuel. Yo-yo dieters might not be familiar with this forgetting-to-eat phenomenon due to a spectacular array of diet rules coupled with food obsession. And if you're currently more tuned into calories or macros than your hunger, you might not even notice surging hunger levels.

Since the emergence of diet culture and the increase in availability of food, we've unlearned the art of listening to our appetites. We've been taught to trust others more than we trust ourselves. By becoming more aware of your hunger, you may be able to get back to this internal body cue so that deciding what and when to eat is far simpler.

Switch off starvation mode

Remember how diets can trigger your body to head into starvation mode, making you hungrier while slowing your metabolism? Well, to get out of starvation mode, your body needs food. Makes sense, right? And it needs to know it's safe to eat without all those niggly restrictions. Eating *ad libitum* (that's a fancy way of saying 'eating when hungry') can help toggle off the survival switch. Eating food freely helps to send a notification to your brain that the famine is over. It can chill. If you've identified that 'eating enough food' is one of your habit gaps, then eating according to your appetite is something that can help.

If you're struggling with diet burnout or even if you're not, practising intuitive eating is a smart thing to do. I highly recommend it!

Intuitive eating

How does intuitive eating work? I'm glad you asked. Do you ever get home and turn into a cookie monster, devouring anything from your child's leftover bread crusts to handfuls and handfuls of nuts, followed by the entire contents of the pantry? A couple of things might be at play here: either it's because cookies are delicious (I'm a big fan) OR there's good chance you're arriving home ravenously hungry.

When you get too hungry (ravenous), you are more likely to turn to sugar and refined carbs for a speedy boost to your energy levels. This may explain why, when you're overly hungry, you don't reach for a salad or an apple but crave higher-energy foods such as cake, peanut butter, cheese, chips or burgers.

Once you're THAT hungry, your body flings itself at anything with calories. This intense hunger can result in binge eating of breads, cereals, peanut butter straight from the jar and chocolate or lollies. Or you may find yourself compulsively eating things like vegetables and fruit. Your ravenous body prefers high-energy foods, but it doesn't discriminate. It'll take what it can get!

It makes sense to try to notice and respond to your rising hunger levels BEFORE you plummet into chaotically eating anything in sight.

There are some useful things to know about your appetite:
* Your hunger tends to gradually build with time.
* Your hunger changes according to factors like the weather, lifestyle, how much you move your body, stress and sleep, etc.
* Your hunger can be predictable, even though it shifts around.

Once you tune into your hunger, you might notice patterns emerging. Many people I've helped would often eat 'in case of hunger'. Being too hungry isn't fun, so recognising your body's own natural hunger patterns may help you sidestep this habit.

For example, I'm not very hungry when I first wake up in the morning. My hunger cues tend to build so that by 10 or 11 am I'm ready to have breakfast. That is when I eat most mornings. Occasionally, I wake up hungry and I'll eat at 7 am when my toddler eats, but this is rare. If I wait until about noon to have my first meal, I'm generally too hungry by then. What I'm saying is, my body has its own rhythm. I get hungry generally around the same time each day, give or take.

What does hunger feel like for you?

My fellow dieters might feel a little confused about hunger. How do you know when you're hungry? After all, diets instruct us to ignore hunger and eat by the clock or according to the meal plan.

Some basic physical sensations that can help you recognise hunger:

* grumble in your stomach
* an 'empty' feeling in your stomach
* hunger 'pangs' or stomach pains
* a weird gut feeling that it's time to eat
* fatigue
* declining concentration
* lightheadedness
* anger
* cranky or feeling edgy
* headache
* feeling shaky

The first four sensations tend to happen at the earlier stages of hunger, while some of the more intense experiences (fatigue and onwards) can happen when you're already quite intensely hungry.

While diets are easy to start, they're hard to follow in the long term. Intuitive eating is the opposite. It can be harder to start, as you need to take time to learn what hunger feels like for you and notice patterns. With just a touch of practice, it's easier to stick to the longer you do it. With time, you'll find you can more seamlessly distinguish when you're hungry or full. And one essential tool to help you do that is the hunger scale.

✎ What does hunger feel like for you?

When you next get hungry, note down the sensations you feel in your body, trying your best to describe the sensation. Do the same thing after you've eaten to help identify what 'fullness' feels like for you.

The hunger scale

The hunger scale is a simple tool that can help you become more acquainted with your innate hunger cues so you can mostly eat when hungry, and stop when you are full. Rating your hunger using the hunger scale may help you get back in touch with your appetite.

It's handy to think of the hunger scale as the fuel gauge of a car. Your appetite is telling you how much fuel your body needs. Think of '0' as empty. No energy left! As you eat food, you refuel your energy tank, filling it back up to be fuller.

By tuning into your hunger, you learn to fuel your body without needing to count macros or points or weigh your food. On the hunger scale, 0 is ravenously hungry while 10, the other extreme, means you feel stuffed full. Ideally, you want your hunger and fullness to swing gently between comfortably hungry and comfortably full, as opposed to swinging between the extremes of too hungry and too full.

Too hungry		Comfortably hungry			Peckish		Comfortably full		Too full	
0	1	2	3	4	5	6	7	8	9	10
Ravenous!	Uncomfortably hungry	Aim to eat		Getting hungry	'I could eat'	Getting full	Aim to stop eating		Uncomfortably full	Stuffed!

✎ Rank your hunger on a scale of 0 to 10

How hungry are you? Practise using the hunger scale to rank your hunger levels right now as you're reading this. What number would you say you are on the hunger scale?

Am I hungry?

A key part of eating intuitively is to ask yourself before eating, 'Am I hungry?' It's the equivalent of Marie Kondo's question, 'Does this spark joy?' Often we eat because it's meal time or we're bored. Asking if you're hungry can help you eat according to your body's energy needs.

A Better Way To Be Healthy

Aim to eat when 'comfortably hungry'

Your tank is getting low, but you still have energy left. This is represented by a two to three on the hunger scale. As with a car, you don't want to wait until you're stalled on the side of a road, coughing and spluttering and having to call in emergency support! You want to eat before you get ravenously hungry or 'hangry'. As you eat, you'll notice the impact eating has on your hunger levels. Hunger will begin to fade and will at some point be replaced with a sense of fullness, or a neutral feeling where hunger is no longer present.

That's when you're so hungry you feel angry, something my husband tells me I have experienced.

Aim to stop eating when 'comfortably full'

In an ideal world, you try to stop eating when you feel 'comfortably full', which is a seven to eight on the hunger scale. This won't always happen. You might still eat until you feel stuffed. As you practise intuitive eating, abandoning those diet rules and trusting that 'anytime I am hungry, I am allowed to eat', you may find it easier to happily stop eating when you reach that comfortably full spot.

Some tips for eating intuitively

* **Eat when you're hungry.** Remind yourself: any time I feel hungry, I am allowed to eat. This is an important thing to take on board if you want to flick off the starvation switch and help your body realise there is no hold-back on food. It can help your body feel that its essential need to 'eat enough food' (Level 1 of the hierarchy) is being satisfied.
* **Notice your patterns.** With time, you'll notice some patterns emerging. Become curious about these patterns and how long it takes you to move from peckish on the hunger scale to 'comfortably hungry'. For example, it may take about one hour to 90 minutes to go from peckish to hungry, which is handy to know so that in the real world, feeling peckish could act as a notification, reminding you to think about getting food soon.
* **Intuitive eating isn't a diet rule.** It's tempting to want to do intuitive eating perfectly! But this isn't yet another diet rule. You don't need to get it right all the time. And you won't. Sometimes there will be seriously delicious chocolate cake that you won't want to miss, so

you'll ending up feeling more full than is comfortable. Likewise, you might forget to eat or have a shift that runs late, meaning you are more hungry than you'd like by the time you eat. This is OK. This is life. Remember, none of us are robots or Rapunzel. Simply aim to become more curious about waxing and waning hunger levels, to eat according to your appetite and then be compassionate and curious when it doesn't happen.

Shameless plug: In my Back to Basics app, I have a hunger check-in tool that helps identify patterns around when you might be getting too hungry or if you are eating until you are too full and gives you some practical strategies around dealing with those pesky times.

Common questions

For frequent dieters, intuitive eating can be a little confusing at first. What does eating according to hunger even look like? Here are some As to some frequently asked Qs.

Q: How do I measure portion size?

A: So many people want to know, 'How much am I ALLOWED to eat?' It's a normal, sensible question for a dieter to ask. After all, the diet world loves to tell us the 'right' amount of food to eat according to metrics such as calories or carbohydrates. This means portion recommendations are NOT based on appetite or fullness or satisfaction.

The right amount of food to eat depends on your hunger. Some days you're going to burn more energy (hello, hungry days) and other days you'll need a bit less energy. Eating until you feel satisfied and waiting until you feel hungry to eat means you don't need to control portion sizes. In fact, controlling portion sizes may be making it harder for you to eat the recommended portion size or you're left with guilt when you eat more than you were told you were supposed to. Plus, it's only adding to your mental load, reducing your willpower reserves.

When you simply tune into your hunger to guide you on how much food your body needs at any given time, it simplifies things. Suddenly, you transform thinking from 'How much am I allowed to eat?' to 'How much do I feel like eating?' It goes from consulting an external 'expert' to returning to your body, the real expert.

A Better Way To Be Healthy

Q: Should I stick to the serving size suggestions on food packages?

A: The back of food packages also have a 'portion size' recommendation. For example, one slice of bread is one portion size. And apparently a chocolate bar contains 2.5 servings, even though it comes in non-resealable packaging. Many dieters read these food labels and assume 'this is how much I'm meant to eat' without realising what the food industry is really playing at. Because I used to work at a food company, and have consulted with many, I know how the game is played.

Serving-size suggestions on the back of a food packet are pure marketing, with the aim of making a food appear better for you than it actually is. Suggesting a smaller portion size allows manufacturers to make us – health-conscious consumers – believe their product contains less sugar, fat or whatever else we've been told to avoid than it actually does. It makes customers more likely to buy it (thanks to the 'health halo' effect). And it may mean a food company can make health claims like 'Less than 100 calories!' or 'Contains less sugar' if the recommended serving size ticks those boxes. Realise that these serving sizes have nothing to do with your appetite or what you should be eating. It's a marketing tactic.

What is the health halo effect?

We get tricked into thinking something is healthier because it's peppered with enticing nutrient claims. Marshmallows were seen as healthy during the nineties because they are 'fat free' (even though they are nearly entirely made of sugar). Himalayan pink salt, compared to normal salt, has tiny amounts of minerals present. It's sold to us as 'healthier' even though it's just expensive salt. Sometimes companies put healthy-ish products in green packaging to trick us into thinking they're healthier than they are.

Q: I've been told to eat every few hours to keep my metabolism going. I also often eat because it's meal time and I want to eat with my family. What should I do?

A: If you've been on restrictive diets, you may have been taught to ignore physical hunger and simply 'eat by the clock' or a meal plan. You might discover there are times when you're eating simply because it's breakfast time, even when you aren't hungry. But if you aren't hungry, you don't need to eat every few hours to keep your metabolism going. Let your hunger, not diet rules, guide you on when is the best time to eat for your body. However, I totally get that you'd want to enjoy dinner with your family! If you find you're having a big afternoon snack because you're ravenous by that point, having more to eat for lunch could be the key. The number one problem I see ex-dieters making is that they don't eat enough during the day because they're 'trying to be good'. Eating more for lunch might mean you don't raid the pantry in the afternoon, helping you feel hungry for family dinner time.

Is breakfast the most important meal of the day?

The idea that breakfast is the most important meal of the day was invented by John Harvey Kellogg. Yes, the same Kellogg who started the famous breakfast cereal brand (not that he was biased or anything). We've also been sold the idea that breakfast is important for weight loss. And yet, research shows that people who don't eat breakfast may weigh less. And adding breakfast to your diet doesn't actually lead to weight loss. Breakfast is a fantastic chance to get some key nutrients like calcium, fibre and protein (often found in wholegrain breakfast cereal with milk or yoghurt, or some fluffy eggs with wholegrain toast). Ultimately, if you're an adult, and you're not hungry when you wake up in the morning, you don't need to force yourself to eat. Simply wait until you do feel hungry to have breakfast, whether that's at 6 am or 11 am.

Q: Why do I have such a big appetite?

A: This is a common phrase I hear from dieters. Maybe you don't have a big appetite. Maybe (and likely) you probably have a perfectly normal appetite for your body. But thanks to meal plans and diet culture, you've been convinced that a measly 1200 calorie diet is enough for a grown woman to function on. You believe eating anything more than that is too much. You compare your natural hunger and appetite to that of a starvation diet (ahem, I mean weight-loss plan). It's no wonder you feel gluttonous, unable to stick to a squirrel-sized portion.

1200 calories is not enough food, by the way. That's how much energy a toddler requires.

Q: Am I allowed to eat more than my partner? Can I have seconds?

A: You are allowed to eat as much or more than your partner! You are allowed to go back for seconds. You are allowed to eat more than the recipe serving suggests. You are allowed to eat potatoes, pasta and rice. Some days you'll find you are hungrier than others and that's OK. You can trust your hunger and your body to help you eat the right amount of energy it needs to feel good. When we try to control what we eat, tell ourselves we 'should only be eating a small portion', it can do funny things to our brain. You might find you think about food more, have more cravings and feel insatiable. But when we accept that our body needs different amounts of food on different days and that our hunger will help guide us to eat the energy we need, we can relax around food. We can finish a meal and move on with our lives, without feeling deprived and preoccupied by food. You might find you don't end up bingeing later in the day. You really are allowed food and allowed to eat as much as your body needs. Even if that's more than what you think you 'should' be eating.

Of course, part of the fun of being human means your appetite can be complex. Lingering diet rules or thoughts like, 'I just ate! Surely I'm not still hungry?' can make listening to your physical hunger a little tricky. Let's explore how these things contribute to emotional hunger.

Emotional hunger

Unlike physical hunger, emotional hunger can come on quite quickly – and it may be all consuming. While physical hunger is satiated when you eat something (almost anything with energy), emotional hunger has quite specific needs. It can explain why you aren't satisfied with a savoury meal until it's been finished off with a bite of something sweet. Interestingly, chronic dieters often deny their emotional hunger, leading to a feeling of restriction. This happens when you say, 'I shouldn't be eating this' or 'If I eat this I'll have to be good tomorrow.' These judgements around food can lead to perpetual, underlying and hard-to-pinpoint emotional hunger.

Emotional hunger can contribute to your body thinking there isn't enough food, even if you have eaten sufficient calories.

The thing is, emotional eating is normal. Everyone does it: it's a standard reaction to stress. After a tough day, you might say, 'I feel like emotional eating', have something to eat, feel better and then move on. I don't think aiming for zero emotional eating is the goal. It only becomes problematic when it happens frequently and there's a sense of feeling out of control. It's worse when you add a side serving of guilt and shame.

Satisfying emotional hunger

The most important thing to start with? Combatting restrictions. That means helping your body realise that no foods are off limits. If you've been dieting for years, you might have a whole bunch of foods that you currently feel are off limits. As such, they seem highly interesting to you, like those participants with the Macaroni and Cheese diet (see page 29) on the first day of the experiment. Continuing to avoid foods you consider 'bad' can only make you feel more out of control around them. As an ex-dieter, it might sound scary but you need to give yourself permission to eat the foods you have been denying yourself, while not beating yourself up for doing it.

Won't that just lead to more out-of-control eating?

You might be worried: 'If I'm allowed to eat these foods, won't I simply lose control around them? Won't I eat them all the time and find I'm not able to stop?' Well, surprisingly, the opposite can happen. If dieting has led you to feel out of control, isn't it interesting to think about what would happen if you did the reverse?

When we start to reintroduce forbidden foods after a long time of dieting, there may be a reset period. The body is still quite excited by these previously forbidden foods. It's like a cow that's been grazing in one pasture for its life. One day, the farmer swings open the gates and lets the cow roam around the whole farm. There are so many new pastures! For a brief period, the cow eats and eats. Until finally the cow realises that they aren't getting moved back into the old pasture. They're staying here, in this better location, for good. They don't need to try to eat as much as they can. The food is not going to run out or suddenly be taken away again. Slowly, their cravings regulate and they go back to being as interested in food as they were before.

A Better Way To Be Healthy

When you first quit dieting, there may be a period of time when you're getting used to the idea that no foods are off limits. After avoiding them for so many years, those foods are probably still going to be wonderfully exciting. 'You mean I can sit at a cafe and eat a flaky almond croissant and NOT feel guilty about it?' or 'I can't believe I'm allowed to eat fresh sourdough whenever I feel like it!' You might go crazy eating them for a period of time. But with time your body learns to trust that those foods truly are allowed. They are normalised. Like the macaroni and cheese being served every day, you realise it's not special. It's just another food. You move on with your life. With time, as your body learns that it can eat what it wants, when it wants, you regain control over food.

The big difference? Instead of needing to avoid fried food because it's 'bad' or 'fattening', you might come to realise that you don't like how you feel when you eat fried food. Instead of feeling like a rule, something you 'should' do, you're able to make CHOICES around food.

There are a whole bunch of reasons to focus on your emotional hunger by eliminating restrictions. And it's a key part of creating a healthy relationship with food.

Satisfaction

How much does mindset really matter when it comes to the food we eat? Does our relationship to food – and our perception of how healthy or unhealthy something is – impact how our body digests food and the hormones that get released?

In an experiment known as the 'milkshake study', researchers made a big batch of a 380 calorie French vanilla milkshake, then split the mixture in two.[1] Half the study participants were given a milkshake that had been poured into a bottle labelled the 'sensible' shake, with claims the drink had zero fat, no added sugar and only 140 calories. The remaining mixture was labelled as an 'indulgent' shake, claimed to contain 620 calories, along with fat and sugar, and given to the remaining study participants.

Blood samples were taken from the participants before and after drinking the shake, to measure their levels of the 'hunger hormone' ghrelin. What is ghrelin? When you haven't eaten for a while, the level of ghrelin builds up and this can make you feel hungry. The more ghrelin, the greater the urge to eat. A higher level of ghrelin also slows your metabolism (in case you can't readily access food). Then, once you've eaten, the ghrelin level drops so that you no longer feel hungry.

Fascinatingly, the ghrelin levels of those who'd drunk the 'indulgent' shake went down three times more than those who had the lighter 'sensible' shake! In fact, those who had the 'sensible' shake had a relatively flat ghrelin response. What does this mean? Your body responds differently to what you eat based on your beliefs about that food.

You see, it's really not just about calories in versus calories out. The way you think about food matters. This means our obsession with labelling every food as 'good' or 'bad' is problematic. It impacts us psychologically and physiologically. Chasing 'clean' or 'sensible' options may not be serving you. It may explain why the low-fat movement failed so many of us. The French seem to understand this. They eat cheese and full-fat options that satisfy rather than trying to include 'healthier' dupes that leave them wanting. Because satisfaction and how food is labelled matters. And your relationship with food not only changes what and how you eat, but also how your body responds to that food.

Bye-bye, food obsession

As long as you are emotionally and/or physically restricting, you will likely find your brain can't stop thinking about food. And this obsession with food can make it harder to eat healthily or eat according to your hunger levels. It sets you up for all-or-nothing thinking about food, yo-yo dieting and being overwhelmed by all the nutrition noise that clouds your brain. It's an exceptionally good idea to address emotional and physical restriction. The end results are lovely.

Guilt won't help you eat less or lose weight. It will give you a sinking pit-of-your-stomach feeling, screw with your happiness, isolate you from the people you love and ruin what's meant to feel awesome. And while we're at it, guilt doesn't help you eat any healthier. It sets you up for all-or-nothing thinking and we all know how that ends, right? Hello undereating that immediately spirals into out-of-control overeating.

Food guilt has ruined many holidays for me. To help me come back to enjoying myself instead of spending the whole trip resenting the hotel buffet or trying to figure out how to lose weight when I get home, I think: 'A few weeks of less-than-perfect eating isn't going to destroy my health' in the same way that a few weeks of perfectly healthy eating won't transform it. When you get back from a holiday of totally relaxing around food and eating lots of fun options, you might find you naturally crave more home-cooked meals and fresh, leafy things. But only if you leave the guilt behind.

Benefits of addressing emotional hunger

✶ It may be easier to make healthy choices that feel good for your body.
✶ You're better able to tune in to your appetite: to eat when you're hungry and stop eating when you're full.
✶ It increases the chance you'll be able to stick to essential health-based diets to treat things like IBS, reflux or intolerances.
✶ You have reduced guilt around food.
✶ You feel more relaxed around food.
✶ Reduction in all-or-nothing thinking.
✶ More headspace to think about other things.
✶ Easier to make food choices.
✶ Reduce or eliminate emotional or binge eating.
✶ Getting more enjoyment from food.
✶ Actually feeling emotionally and physically satisfied after you eat.
✶ You may no longer feel 'addicted' to food.
✶ It will help you feel less obsessed with food.

Hormonal hunger

Your hormones have a huge impact on your hunger levels. They really run the show. If you're not getting enough shut-eye or you're stressed out all the time, it can lead to an insatiable hunger. Becoming aware of some of the little things that influence your hormones, and understanding their impact on your hunger, may help you better listen and respond to your body.

Sleep

Sleep is the key foundation of health. And yet, many of us underestimate how lack of sleep can significantly impact hunger hormones and lead to a surge in appetite. Combine poor-quality sleep with high stress levels, and it might explain why your cravings for high-energy food feel so intense. This is one of the reasons why sleep is an essential habit! If you aren't refuelling your body with sleep, it may seek out energy in chocolate form when reserves get low after a gruelling day. If you're looking to get healthier, prioritising good-quality sleep is important.

Your hunger levels are actually controlled by a bunch of body chemicals, called neurotransmitters. When you skip quality sleep, you may actually feel more hungry – and it's not just your imagination. People who are sleep deprived have higher levels of the hunger hormone ghrelin and inhibited levels of leptin, the hormone that helps you feel satisfied after eating.[2] Along with the fact that different brain regions are affected by how much sleep you get, this means that people who don't get enough sleep tend to consume more energy.[3]

It's not just your eating that crappy sleep is impacting. Poor sleep affects your immune system and impacts your body's ability to recover. It can affect energy levels and how sociable you feel like being. And it has a big impact on your mood. After all, there is a reason why sleep deprivation has been used as a torture device.[4]

A study from Norway showed that interrupted or poor-quality sleep affected 50 to 80 per cent of mental health patients.[5] It used to be assumed that bad sleep was a symptom of mood disorders, but what it is most like is a bidirectional relationship[6] – a bit of a chicken or egg situation. Not enough sleep can put you at risk of developing mood disorder and having a mood disorder may mean you don't get enough sleep. Then consider how your eating changes when your mood isn't in the best place, further adding to this whole food situation!

Stress

When you're stressed, levels of the stress hormone cortisol increase. And cortisol can increase appetite and change how fat is stored in your body. But stress can also show in the body in a number of other ways. For one, it can cause skin reactions like eczema or your gut to become upset, leading to unpleasant bowel movements. There is a tendency to

A Better Way To Be Healthy

misdiagnose food intolerances, assuming gluten or dairy are to blame when stress can be a big contributor. Stress may also result in your drinking more alcohol, a depressive substance. That may help explain why you have a bad case of 'hanxiety' the day after drinking too much.

Another thing that can cause stress in the body, beyond annoying emails and the sound of a child crying? Undereating. And over-exercising. While exercise can help combat stress (and those pesky high cortisol levels) by releasing endorphins and helping you sleep better at night, overdoing it can place your body under physical stress. The result is cortisol being released into your bloodstream. It's also important to note that undereating and overexercising can be the way some people respond to stressful situations. This is why we'll talk more about stress management, another core habit, in Chapter 9.

Menstrual cycle

You're not imagining it, my friend. Some days it's easier to be confident or fall asleep or manage your cravings. Some days are better than others for going swimwear shopping or taking a photo you like. Some days are perfect for making plans while other days (I learned the hard way) work out best when you make no plans at all. I discovered all of this and heaps more by tracking my period for nine months. Yes, it was a slightly weird thing to do. I surprised myself! Yet, I'd do it all again because what I've learned has transformed how I live – and my health.

I was holidaying in the south of Spain. (Amazing, right? If only it had felt that way.) I should have been feeling fabulous, but my mood and confidence were low. I felt bloated and emotional. All of this stopped me from being able to have fun or feel confident. But just two weeks earlier, I had been feeling wonderful, sexy and energetic! So I checked the date, and sure enough, my period was days away.

Could my period be having such big impact on my life, and I'd just never realised? You see, I'd spent the previous two decades thinking my period was a burden. In fact, I tried not to think about my period at all! Except at times when it embarrassed me. Like when I had to shove tampons down my sleeve to go to the bathroom at work. Or when my period caught me unawares (as has happened to all of us). Here I was, finally realising that maybe my period was worth paying attention to. Could understanding my period help me take care of my body?

Here's what I learned. There are four phases of the menstrual cycle. This is based on fluctuating hormones. Learning how you can work with the hormonal shifts, rather than against them, can help you know yourself better. You may even be able to predict how you'll feel.

And so with a healthy dose of scepticism – and curiosity about the science behind it all – I began tracking my cycle. I'd tried to use apps before, but found the habit never stuck. So this time, I just started tracking my cycle in a calendar app on my computer. I didn't intend to track it daily or for nine months but, driven by curiosity, it just happened. It was a very quick, imperfect process so I got it done without overthinking it.

Every day, I'd note which day of my cycle I was on (e.g. Day 1 or Day 28) and then I'd record how the following things were going for me: mood, body confidence, skin, hunger and cravings, exercise, bowel movements, sleep and sex drive. Here's what I learned. The week before my period, a whole lot of important shifts may happen. I noticed that my body confidence took a nose dive. The temptation to diet was very strong at this time (even starting from day 18). I felt more bloated and I rated my body as looking softer. If you weigh yourself

✎ Get to know your cycle

If you menstruate, you might want to track it for yourself. I wonder if it's the same for you, how your period influences your body confidence, desire to diet, hunger, cravings, sleep and more. Research suggests it's all connected.[7] Consider tracking your period for one month to see what changes happen for you. It can be a very interesting experiment!

Here's how you do it: use a paper diary or a digital calendar (like I did), work out what day of your cycle you're currently on. Day 1 is the first day of your period. Depending on your cycle length, start mapping out your cycle. Each day, add a quick note recording how you feel about your mood, body confidence, skin, hunger and cravings, exercise, bowels, sleep and sex drive. Or add different categories depending on your goals.

After a month of insights, you'll already start to get a sense of just how your menstrual cycle influences many facets of your health.

during this time, you might find a 0.3–1 kilogram (0.7–2.2 lb) weight gain due to water retention.

For me, simply realising, 'It's OK, you tend to feel unhappy with your body around this week. It's not your body, it's your hormones. Wait until next week and see how you feel' has prevented me from attempting many quick fixes and is another way that I am actively kind to myself. Once my period comes, my body confidence flourishes again. And I'm back to my normal body-accepting self.

It's common to feel pre-period food cravings. 'WHERE IS THE CHOCOLATE?' written in shouty caps is pretty much me the week before my period. Some research suggests an increase in the number of cravings in the days leading up to a period by up to 66 per cent.[8] You may eat more or feel a touch more depressed and it's all thanks to those surging hormones.

Why? People experience changing levels of four different hormones throughout their cycles. They tend to crave higher-energy food before their period and they might notice hunger reducing again from Day 1 of their cycle.

Day 1 is the first day of your period, by the way.

For me, cravings are high but what I notice most is that I am noticeably hungrier. So I don't fight it. When my hunger increases, I trust that my body needs more food. I respond by feeding it more, without judgement.

Here's the thing. If you keep fighting against this increase in hunger or boost in cravings, and keep trying to push on even though you feel more tired and moody than usual, you're telling your body you're not listening. You might blame yourself for having an 'insatiable appetite', thinking it's a personal flaw when it's really just a natural bodily process.

If you're unaware of this increase in hunger, and still stuck on a meal plan trying to eat the same thing you usually do, you might find it's even harder to diet during the pre-period week. Meal plans tell you to eat the same thing every day because, for people who don't have periods, this might be more doable. For those whose sex hormones oscillate within a 28-day cycle, it's very handy to work with your hormonal fluctuations, not against them.

Though the research suggests it's not doable for them either.

During ovulation (so Day 14-ish of the cycle), your hunger may decrease. And if you were ever to 'forget to eat', it may be around this time of the month. What tracking your menstrual cycle teaches you is that there is no need to fight your body. Your body is guiding you – sometimes it's more hungry, sometimes it's less – and you simply need to practise listening to it.

Knowing that your physical hunger will naturally change during the month as your hormones surge may help you to eat more in tune with your body's needs. Some weeks you will be ravenous, others you might find you forget to eat. Learning to be OK with the changes can help you feel more calm around food so you can finally stop dieting or stressing about your weight for good.

Perimenopause

During the years leading up to and through menopause, hunger levels will also likely increase as your hunger hormone ghrelin goes up. At the same time, leptin, the hormone that helps you feel full, can be reduced. This can explain why you suddenly feel hungrier than you can remember being before. This is on top of random hair growth and the fact that your cravings for yummy things are probably spiking too. It's a wild ride (so I've heard). What to do about it? Prioritising sleep is a biggie during this time. And I know, I know. That too can be harder to find thanks to the sweatiness and heart-rate changes. The number one thing to do is avoid the temptation to diet. Because your metabolism shifts during this time, it can be a tricky time for body image too. The same sound advice is still the best approach, which means listening to your body, being kind to yourself and adopting healthy habits, not crash dieting.[8]

Why do hormones matter?

Many things impact your hormonal hunger – from how much sleep you get, to stress levels and cycling sex hormones during your menstrual phase or perimenopause – causing dips and dives, and resulting in your body storing energy as fat differently. Beyond the physical grumble in your stomach kind of hunger, hormones really impact on your baseline hunger levels. Of course, then your emotional hunger – that is, how you feel and think about food – adds another layer to how hunger walks. Your body has many biological processes in place to ensure you eat enough food and feel rested. It doesn't care if you don't have a thigh gap or lean, non-jiggly arms. It just wants you to be healthy. And while you might think your conscious brain is in control, your body's calling the shots. That's lucky, really. Because even if you don't love your body yet, your body already loves you. It's programmed to protect you. So it's time to stop fighting against your body and start working with it to be healthy, even if that means not looking perfect.

Even if you don't love your body yet, your body already loves you.

Essential takeaways

* **Physical hunger:** Practise tuning in to your hunger using the hunger scale. Can you wait until you feel hungry to eat instead of eating just because you normally do or because it's meal time? Can you notice rising hunger levels and remind yourself you can always eat more food whenever you need? You can use my Back to Basics app to help you record your hunger.
* **Emotional hunger:** Working to break down lingering food rules will help you reduce the intensity of emotional hunger to more manageable levels (like that of someone who has never dieted).
* **Hormonal hunger:** Do not underestimate the power of sleep, hormones and stress and how they can influence hunger, mood, energy, immunity and a bunch of other things. With female hormonal fluctuations, can you start to notice and work with those changes instead of fighting against them, insisting on functioning the same every day, even though you feel completely different on day 14 versus day 28 of your cycle?

Chapter 9.

Managing stress

Unmanaged stress may impact on our quality of sleep, how much we eat or how we feel about ourselves. Prioritising rest and self-care may help combat the negative impacts of some stress, which is why it's a core habit in Level 2 of the hierarchy of healthy habits. But even if we know rest is something we absolutely require for our health and mental wellbeing, a bunch of things can stop us from taking the time we need to recharge.

It took me seven weeks from the time I got a prescription from my doctor for eczema cream (a flare-up is a warning signal from my body when I'm too stressed and run down) to the time I got the ointment from the pharmacy. Seven weeks of 'it can wait until tomorrow'; 'it's not THAT bad'; 'there are more important things in my life than me'; and 'I'm too busy'. And my eczema got worse.

Eventually, I couldn't ignore it anymore. By then, my knees were bleeding and a furry circular patch of hair had sprouted around them. The area was too sensitive to shave but, realistically, shaving was pretty low on my priority list anyway. So there I was with furry, bleeding knees, but at least my house was vacuumed and unsolicited messages from random people had been responded to, right?

Ah-ha! I see. I'm not the priority in my own life. That's what I realised after the furry-bleeding-knee debacle. If my son or husband – or even my dog – needed medication, I would have bought it the same day the doctor gave me the prescription. Everyone is more important than me. I sacrifice my physical and mental health for other things. I'll give up my energy to strangers or use up valuable time wondering about that aggressive driver and whether I really offended them that much, instead of realising they were just in a shit mood.

How to be kind to yourself

I used to be pretty good at beating myself up. I'd lie in bed at night for hours running over all the ways I'd ever failed (there are lots!) but neglecting the ways I'd done good.

I expect a lot from myself. And so I'd get disappointed when I'm anything less than perfect. But that way of living was ruining me.

I couldn't keep ruining holidays and happy memories by being so harsh on myself. So now my goal is simple. Be kind to myself. Not just normal kind. Incredibly kind. As in . . . exceptionally kind. This meant changing my thought patterns and default habits.

What I realised is that when I am kind to myself, I am so much more confident. I no longer rely on compliments from others to feel good. Because I'm kind to myself, I don't feel tied to other people's opinions. I care less about what other people think. I love (or at least accept) my body more. And it feels fantastic.

You don't have to love yourself. That's a lot of pressure. But you may find it'll come from being kinder to yourself. Being kind is the act; the result is loving yourself. So start with the act and the feeling will follow. Being kind to yourself isn't something you just wake up and magically do one morning. It's a process. It's something you have to actively choose to do every day.

Being kind to yourself looks like:

* forgiving yourself for not being perfect
* choosing to remind yourself that you are already enough. Even when your brain insists you are inadequate.
* focusing on your best qualities, rather than your shortcomings
* saying 'no' when people ask too much of you (the temporary discomfort you might experience is far better than resenting them or yourself later because you said 'yes')

Constant self-improvement

I'll be honest. I love a self-help book. I've bought tonnes of them during my life, and what do you know, it seems I'm writing one right now. But at what point does all this self-optimising become harmful?

The reason we dive into advice about how to improve our lives is fundamentally that we don't feel good enough as we are. So if we try this or do that thingamajig, maybe we'd stop feeling like we're failing.

Sometimes I feel like I spend my entire life cleaning my house. But I've realised the cleaning never ends. By the time I've done all my

Rage cleaning. It's a thing.

Recently, I've got a new, um . . . hobby. Rage cleaning. Rage cleaning is the act of frantically cleaning your home while fuming at the fact that no one offers to help. The rage sears inside you, making you more and more angry with each swipe or sweep. 'Fine, I'll do it myself!' you yell to no one in particular. Or you slam the cabinet door violently to alert others to the fact that you are cleaning alone! Again! Why do I bother creating a chore chart?

The whole time I'm cleaning, I'm ruminating about how I should ask for help, while never actually asking for help. When help is finally offered, the anger is too deep, so I sigh theatrically and refuse. 'Argh. You left me to clean for this long. I'm going to finish the job myself. You don't get to win.'

And if I do let them help me out with the cleaning, it probably won't be for very long as they're not doing a good enough job anyway, so I'll have to come back and do it again, so I may as well have just done it in the first place and how come you can be so smart and do our taxes but you can't remove the lint from the dryer filter?

Rage cleaning. Maybe you're familiar? It also tends to come with a hearty helping of guilt and stress. I need to learn to be kinder to myself.

to-do list tasks, the original ones need to be redone again. At what point do I get to relax, arrive at my clean-house destination and enjoy it? A rigorous house-cleaning schedule can promise to help you feel more calm in your space. But at what point does it stop being something helpful and become something we compulsively need to keep up with, yet another ball to keep in the air? Like the way your email inbox will never be empty, maybe your house will never be perfectly clean. And your body may never be the perfectly acceptable size.

Keeping your house clean is an impermanent state. Just like being in a calorie deficit. It takes a hell of a lot of work to maintain something just for the day, and then the next day you have to do it all over again. It's fundamentally about control and avoiding discomfort. It's just one way perfectionism can take over our lives. When the rigid standards that have been set for us by others or by ourselves interfere with our wellbeing, physical or mental.

If we don't lower our crushing standards, and decide that things can be a bit more jumbled and imperfect than we'd like, we may be miserable forever. Do you ever feel like you're just existing? Living, yes. For sure. But sometimes it's like you're just sleeping and eating and working and repeating (along with some cleaning and laundry). It can feel like you're just planning your life but never really existing inside it. Too busy taking care of everyone else to care for yourself. But never quite getting to the dream destination.

There's a big problem with trying to control or hack or optimise every moment of being. It closes you off to potential opportunities. When you're so hyper-focused on specific goals, you miss out on the opportunities. Like those science experiments where you're asked to watch a video and count how many times the gymnast does a flip. Only you get to the end of the video and it's revealed that a person in a gorilla suit walked through the video clip. But because your brain was so hyper-focused on what you were trying to achieve, you missed out on the other, more interesting thing.

This happens with food and weight all the time. You get so focused on trying to lose weight, at some point you forget that this thing was meant to be making you happy, giving you more life, not filling your brain with how many almonds you ate that day.

When you're in a natural state of flow, it's kinda wondrous how things tend to follow on from that. You speak to the right person, watch something and then, suddenly, things start falling into place. There is a certain magic (a word I don't use often) to surrendering from the rigid plan and becoming open minded to what could happen.

During my quest for self-love – well, at least self-acceptance – people often told me to 'talk to yourself like you're talking to your best friend'. To be honest? I've always found that advice tricky to implement. I wanted something more practical. So I went looking. And here's what I learned from choosing to be kind to myself.

You can be anything, but you can't be everyone

When scrolling on social media, I see so many different archetypes I want to be. There's the cool and confident woman who has hectically good street style, the wholesome mother playing with her kids in a veggie garden, the career woman winning accolades, the serene person with the perfect-looking home. After years of aspiring to become an amalgamation of these people, at some point I realised what should have been so very obvious: they are not the same people. You can be anything, but you can't be everyone. You can excel in specific domains in life, but not all of them. Striving to achieve it all can often leave you feeling like you're failing across the board. In different seasons of your life, you will play to the different identities you aspire to be. And that's OK. Be who you are right now, be present with yourself and accept that you're choosing to be the best version of your chosen direction.

Ask: 'What can this teach me?'

When you mess up, it can feel easy to beat yourself up with, 'You've ruined it again. What a waste! Now you have to start again.' But messing up – or being imperfect (aka human) – is never a waste of time. Because there is always something to be gained or learned from it. When you next screw up, or find yourself in an uncomfortable situation, ask yourself: 'What can I learn from this?' You'll start to see that nothing is really ruined or a waste of time; for example, sitting in traffic can help teach you patience. An episode of binge eating isn't a failure if you consider that it may reveal what led to the out-of-control pantry raid preventing future bingeing. Every (well, almost every) situation can teach you something.

I like to write things down. It helps get the thought out of my head. Once it's on paper, it feels like closure. Hello, journal that sits next to my bed.

Make your own lunch first

We've talked before about expectations that you will please others before yourself. Many parents make their family members lunch to take to school or work but don't make anything for themselves. My client Amelia had this challenge to overcome. She'd make everyone else in the household a wholesome lunch, but didn't make something for herself to eat. By lunchtime, she'd be hungry and without a prepared meal, so she ended up searching in the pantry for biscuits, or lollies, only to end up overeating at dinner because she was famished by then.

The first hurdle for her was getting over the idea that she needed to eat a salad for lunch. While nutritious and delicious (with yummy dressing and fun ingredients, of course), it's not what she felt like eating. I worked with her on crushing the outdated idea that she wasn't allowed to eat bread or that it was somehow 'bad'.

As a result, she started making herself a sandwich when she made the rest of the family's lunches. How doable. She now had something that genuinely excited her when she got hungry around lunchtime. Because she ditched the idea that bread was 'bad', she ended up having a deliciously satisfying sandwich in place of biscuits and lollies and found she was way more satisfied, so wasn't as hungry by dinnertime. No more emotional or physical restriction meant she was finally eating enough. In the health hierarchy, you don't have to be a nutritionist to understand that a sandwich trumps lollies and biscuits in the health stakes, so this move was a major win.

I've also started doing this, a little act to take care of my future. When I pack my son's lunchbox, I also put some of the same foods aside so I'll have a snack pack ready to go later. As a woman, and as a mother, I really have to fight the temptation to take care of everyone else, neglecting myself. It's really important that you prioritise feeding yourself nutritious food, just as you try to feed your family. Here's my challenge for you: when you are next making food for the family, make your food first – or at least at the same time – and then provide for others.

You're never too old for a snack pack, I've discovered!

If you aren't ready to make drastic life changes, start small. Instead of saying yes to dinner with someone who spends the entire night talking about themselves, suggest a 30 minute coffee catch-up instead. Sure, it might feel uncomfortable at first. But ultimately, the discomfort of saying no is better than resenting it later. Chances are, your friend will be totally fine with it, and you will get 90 minutes of your life back.

Another option? Just give them a mirror so they can be narcissistic with their favourite person.

If you're ensuring everyone else's basic needs are met but not your own, it's time to change. It's time to give to yourself as you give to others. Yes, I'm telling you to put your oxygen mask on first. But, more practically, make your sandwich first. Or at least, make it a priority to give the same attention to yourself as you give to others.

I'm not telling you to be selfish. Just reminding you that you're allowed to take up space, to ask for your fair share and be incredibly kind to yourself.

A Better Way To Be Healthy

What things do you currently do to take care of your future? This isn't meant to feel like one more thing to add to your already out-of-control to-do list, but rather it's something that feels like taking time for yourself.

Some small things I try to do to take care of future me:
* Take off my make-up before bed.
* Drink a glass of water before bed if I drank too much alcohol.
* Moving clothes that don't currently fit me to a different section of the cupboard.
* Scheduling time for me to exercise.

Recognise your social currency

After I gave birth to my son, I went through what felt like an identity crisis, a transformation period that is sometimes called matrescence. I mourned for the person I had once been: younger, more carefree and spontaneous. But I also mourned for the way I used to look. As women, we're taught from a scarily young age that our social value is based on our looks. So, attempting to make myself feel worthy, in my younger years, I'd spent hours each week trying to subscribe to the beauty ideals. Once I became a mother, my free time – the time I would have spent on altering my appearance – had evaporated. So not only was I mourning the loss of time and freedom, but I was coming to terms with the fact that I couldn't keep relying on altering my appearance as a way of feeling worthy. I didn't have the time or energy to pursue it as I once had. But there was real freedom in this. As you age and your looks change, your social currency changes too. Instead of asking, 'How can I change myself so that I can appear valuable to others?', the new question I needed to ask myself was 'What changes do I need to make that will be valuable to me?'

Taming your inner critic

Waiting until you're doing well and feeling good to be kind to yourself is like only watering a plant when it's flowering. Of course, that plant wouldn't survive in the real world and you wouldn't expect it to. An underfed, underloved plant is going to wilt and die.

My client Trish finds it easy to get stuck with her inner critic dictating her mood. 'I loathe what I see in the mirror and call myself horrible names when I feel I've gained weight. These mental demons have ruled my life and it's exhausting, depressing. My life is going by while I'm hiding away and not living all because I have to be a certain size to be "enough" or loved.'

The first step? Realise when you're giving yourself a hard time. If you don't even realise when you're beating yourself up, it's really hard to change. When I lie in bed at night now, and a negative thought comes into my head, I simply try to notice it. I might say to myself, 'Oh, this is a comparison' or 'this is anxiety'. See how I try to separate the emotion from me: I think, 'This is a comparison' rather than 'you are comparing'. I try not to lurch into, 'Oh Lyndi, you're comparing yourself again. Stop it! You've been awake for hours already. You need to sleep!' because that's not very kind. And it doesn't help. This other way is surprisingly simple and wonderfully powerful.

When I notice negative thoughts circling in my head, I actively switch to my mother's voice. This is a kind, soothing voice that says, 'It's okay, you did your best.' Find your mother's voice (or that of another person in your life who always encourages you and helps you keep perspective) and use it often. Perspective is everything. Remind yourself that it's not your job to be perfect from every angle. You are made for grander and more impressive things.

Don't assume you're the problem

If someone is rude to you, is it your default to assume you've done something wrong? Do you think, 'They obviously don't like me; maybe it was something I said?' We often assume fault in these kinds of situations. The truth is, you don't know what they're thinking or what's going on in their life and the far more likely scenario is that it's nothing to do with you. Be self-aware – sure – but also practise giving less shits about what other people (may or may not) think about you. If someone doesn't like you, that's OK. It's not your job to be liked by everyone.

Think of yourself as a magnet. You attract people with the same force that you repel others with. So if you dilute yourself to be more liked by others, you may end up diluting the force with which you attract 'your people' to you.

It's not your purpose in life to look perfect from every angle or to be liked by everyone.

Remind yourself what brings you joy

Sometimes we get so good at pleasing others that we forget we're allowed to have our own opinions and preferences. In order to set healthy boundaries, get curious about what makes you happy and what doesn't. Spend a day asking yourself if you like/enjoy/agree with the things you do, see or hear. Try not to put any judgement behind it. Just notice if your mind or body feels open or closed to it. If you normally agree with your partner or a friend because 'it's easier', take a moment to really think about what you want.

Here's an example of what I figured out:
* I don't like watching scary films. I'd prefer to read a book.
* Being busy all the time makes me feel depleted.
* I'd rather spend time with my friend in person than text or keep up with a group chat.
* Being on social media makes me feel anxious and not good enough.

You may be surprised by what doesn't bring you joy, which will help you get clearer on what actually does. It's liberating to finally be aware of how draining it feels when your actions or words don't align with what you actually believe. And once you start noticing when things don't feel 'right', it'll be hard to ignore. The next time someone asks you what movie you want to watch, what you feel like eating or whether you have spare time, you can speak up instead of responding with 'I don't know, whatever you want'. Try it!

Ask: 'What's the worst that can happen?'

I'm not a superstitious person. If you're not either, hear me out. Write down the worst thing that could happen if you do X.

For example, what's the worst that can happen if:
* I tell my boss I believe I deserve a promotion.
    → I don't get the promotion.

* I finally sign up for that beginner hip-hop class.
  → I seriously suck at dancing hip-hop.
* I don't send that chainmail to 15 of my closest friends.
  → Nothing will happen; no one will die.

Now – is it really that bad? If it is that bad, then of course reconsider. But chances are it won't be as bad as the worst case scenario.

Practise until it becomes a habit

If something is worth fighting for, chances are it's not going to be easy. Being courageous is a habit. And it's still something I struggle with every day. Sometimes, I'm so overwhelmed by how much still needs to change in the wellness industry that I contemplate moving to Costa Rica and raising a family of sloths (true story). So when life gets overwhelming, take a step back, get some clarity, seek out the help you need, and get back on the proverbial horse even if that is for a deep sleep. Because by practising courage, you are putting your desires first, and lighting the way for the dreams of those around you. And that's worth a few dislikes.

Keen to learn more? I've created a list of my favourite books on this topic and more. To get the reading list, head to my website to download it for free: *lyndicohen.com/bookresources.*

Revenge procrastination

This is a thing that happens to busy working professionals or parents. It's when you don't want to go to bed because that's your only pocket of 'free time', the glorious gap before the work and mental load of the following day begins. Are you doing this?

Prioritise real rest

Rest isn't watching TV while writing to-do lists or doomscrolling on social media. It's not a weekend spent at home, reorganising your house in an attempt to bring order to a life that feels chaotic. We need something more concrete.

You have to decide you deserve rest. You can't just take a bath while running through your shopping list. You can't go away on holiday with the family, but spend the whole time cleaning up after everyone. You've got to decide that you're more important than making the bed, responding to an email or vacuuming.

Rest is letting yourself off the hook, truly allowing yourself to do nothing. 'But I can't rest. I'm a parent. I have a job. Responsibilities.' If you feel this way, then it points to the very problem: a belief that taking rest is possible for others but not for you. You can rest. You are allowed to rest. But also, you should rest, for a gajillion reasons. That said, if you're high-functioning or a care-taker, then rest will need to look different for you.

Filling the void of free time

When you finally do get free time, it turns out that what you choose to fill that time with really matters. We have choices. And then there are practical things to consider: it's much easier to open social media and scroll for five minutes (which turns into an hour) between tasks. Or get lost in front of the TV to help disconnect from a turbulent day. The problem is what this does to your brain.

It's harder to spend our free time doing stuff that helps us feel more like ourselves. I'm not talking about being productive in our free time. That's counterproductive. But if we do more things that make us feel like us, a 'lit up' version of ourselves, compared with the numbed out version of ourselves, then that's great.

Try this: next time you're in a waiting room, instead of pulling out your phone for mindless scrolling, can you simply sit there? Use that time to ponder, to be with yourself. Choose not to fill the void, not to create a further void between you and yourself.

Dolce far niente is a well-known Italian phrase that translates as 'the sweetness of doing nothing'. Instead of saying 'I didn't do anything', how about:

* I rested
* I chose to create space
* I practised saying no
* I was still

Lowering your expectations and standards

Chances are you expect yourself to be able to do it all: have an amazing career, the best relationships, a beautiful home, a perfect body and so on. If you're a parent, add: protect your children, give them a safe environment, reduce screen time, entertain, nourish and comfort, all while looking after yourself and maybe also a household or job.

Of course you can't do all of these things and meet all these needs. Guilt may be a by-product of not having enough support around you. It's a symptom of expecting that you are meant to do it all. You do not and, in fact, you cannot.

Guilt for not doing enough

When you feel guilt, you're blaming yourself for not being or doing enough. You're expecting that you can be and do everything you need. You're trying to be an entire village when you're one single person. And guess what that leads to? Burnout.

Instead of wallowing in guilt, consider this. What if guilt is actually a little notification from your body that things need to change? It could be a clue that you need extra support in your life. So when you notice guilt (and that bitchy inner critic pipes up), instead of blaming yourself, pointing out your shortcomings, ask yourself: What support do I need right now?

Wallowing not recommended: there are more fun things to do.

There are two choices: keep rolling around in bed with guilt – that'll leave you feeling vulnerable and not good enough – or see guilt as an opportunity.

What support do you need?

If you had more support, would you be able to do the things you're aiming to do? Some support options:

* Psychologist
* Parents or mothers' group
* Cleaner
* Nanny
* More sleep
* A hug or more touch

- ✸ Someone to walk with
- ✸ Someone to exercise with
- ✸ Some guidance
- ✸ More structure
- ✸ Less structure
- ✸ A dog walker

Let's look at a few examples of how you might find support.

Concern: I don't take my dog for enough walks. I'm a bad carer.
Solution: Sounds like you are a concerned, caring dog companion but guilt is knocking at your door. Hire a dog walker; ask your community group if anyone wants a companion dog to take on walks; arrange for play time with a neighbour's dog.

Concern: I'm not present when I'm with my kids. I'm too tired and I just need time for me.
Solution: 'Thank you, guilt, for alerting me that I'm not lacking, my support structure is!' Ask a friend at your mothers' group to look after your child and then do the same for them so you both get more 'me time'. Ask your partner to take over bath/bedtime so you have time each day to decompress.

Concern: Everything feels overwhelming and too hard.
Solution: Find someone to talk to. No, I don't necessarily mean your mum, or your best friend, or your hairdresser. I mean a professional, who is paid to listen. To give feedback based on evidence. Some people get massages when they're feeling down, but I see a counsellor and it's one of the kindest things I do for myself.

Notice the urge to retreat (or run!)

I love massages and day spas as much as the next person. But it's not really fixing the underlying problem that I'm overstretched and undersupported. Notice the urge to retreat, flee from your life. Going on a retreat isn't fixing the problem. It's fun. It's enjoyable. But you still come back to your old life with the same problems.

One in, one out policy

You can't do lots of things well. Pick the priorities and work on those things. You only have capacity to keep a certain number of plates spinning at the same time. Trying to take on too many new habits is setting yourself up for failure. Balance is not about adding more, it's about sacrificing what you are willing to live without so you can feel better. You need to remove things from your life to find balance. You can't keep adding more things, doing more things, until the plates all come crashing to the floor. If you want to add a new habit, you may need to let go of something else – an old goal or unhelpful mindset – to make it become a reality.

Cut out everything extra

This funny thing happens when we reach burnout. In an attempt to recover, to stop feeling so effing tired all the time, we might google some solutions. Have a bath, one article suggests. Go on holiday. A face mask, perhaps? These are all well and good, but if you have reached burnout-level fatigue, a soak in the tub or a short little weekend away isn't going to cut it. Adding more things to your to-do list, even if it is self-care, isn't going to help.

✎ Reprioritise what is essential

Write a list of all the tasks you absolutely need to do. Then let's write a list of the 'nice to have'. And then a third, 'dream life' list. Here's mine:

Essential	Nice to have	Dream life
✳ Brush teeth	✳ Make the bed	✳ Eat a salad sandwich for lunch and give the kids healthy, home-cooked meals
✳ Feed children/self	✳ Vacuum	
✳ Dress child/self	✳ Eat something that feels good	
✳ Eat food	✳ Brush hair	✳ Have a perfectly clean home all the time
		✳ Be stylishly dressed
		✳ Ensure my children's clothes are matching

A Better Way To Be Healthy

Looking at the list of the 'dream life', it's easier to see how we're falling short. It's no wonder I can't manage to be all those people/things at all times/ever.

Accept what you can't control

When I had a newborn, I accepted that it was going to be hard. Everyone had warned me. And when it wasn't as hard as I thought it was going to be, I felt really relieved. A little smug, if I'm honest. But somewhere along the way, I assumed it'd get easier. There are fewer people telling you how hard it is having a ten-month-old baby and working full time, while trying to do all the things. No one is dropping off casseroles. No one is sending check-in messages. The workload gets bigger. Because I assumed it would get easier, when it wasn't I blamed myself. I thought, 'If I could just do this then I'll start to feel better'.

But maybe that's not the solution at all. You stop feeling like you're failing all the time when you accept how hard it is. This is meant to be hard. It doesn't matter how much I try to fix it, to plan around it, it's going to be hard. And then I can give myself a break, surrender to the things I can't control and accept.

Accepting that it might not get easier, or that you might not be able to solve the problem, is the hardest yet most important part.

If you feel like, 'I am exhausted all the time. I keep trying to fix things. I want life to feel easier,' then perhaps, just maybe, you simply need to accept that it's going to be hard for now. That it will eventually get easier, but what you're going through right now IS tough.

Accept and ask for help

I got COVID-19 at the same time as my one-year-old son, while my partner was overseas. We had to isolate while I was the only parent to do every shift, without being able to leave the front door. Regardless, I did 8000 steps each day simply running after him and our needy puppy-ish golden retriever while I was sick, depleted and overtired. The 'baby' was waking every 30 minutes so the days and nights were long. In short, I wasn't OK. I cried a lot that week, frantically cleaning the house to try to feel like I had some sense of control in a situation when I had absolutely none.

I'm pretty rubbish at asking for help. Even though I enjoy helping others, I feel deeply uncomfortable when someone offers to help me or jumps in to support me. My natural default is to refuse politely and assure them I can do it myself. But just because you CAN do it by yourself (you're a very capable person, this is true), doesn't mean you SHOULD do it by yourself.

I reached out to a very lovely colleague, writer and podcaster Bek Day, a mum of three whose advice was exactly what I needed to be reminded of. Her instructions were clear:

1.   Say yes when someone offers help.
2.   Let your house be messy.

This advice saved me. Lowering my standards while simultaneously being OK with receiving help allowed me to get through.

It's helpful to understand that humans have an inbuilt desire to help. There's something we call the 'helper's high', a mix of brain chemicals (including boosting oxytocin, dopamine and serotonin) that are released when we help someone, making us feel all warm and fuzzy inside.

And this desire to help may be in our make-up as human beings. Toddlers in their second year in life, before they've been programmed to be nice, want to help.[1] Here's how an experiment to test this was set up. A researcher begins to hang little towels on a clothes horse. After the third towel, they drop the peg 'accidentally'. 'Oh no, I've dropped the clothes peg! My clothes peg!' they say, while trying to grab the clothes peg but pretending to be unable to. Seventy per cent of the time, a toddler sees that someone needs help, grabs the clothes peg and passes it to the researcher. They are driven to help.

What's interesting is in the control condition, when the clothes peg on the floor isn't demonstrated as a problem by the researcher, a toddler will rarely pick up the clothes peg.

When people know we need their help, they want to help. It's in our nature to help people in need. But if no one knows we need help, the same helper's high can't be activated. Often we are waiting for someone to come help us, hoping they will guess what we need.

What are we really achieving by pretending to be OK, to have it sorted, when we don't?

Can we be brave and ask for help? Can we stop expecting people to guess we need something when we don't tell them; when we don't ask, or don't appear to be in need of their support?

There is no shame in having a mental illness

Whispering about mental illness isn't protecting the person you're talking about. It perpetuates the idea that it's not OK to not be OK. We do not need to talk in muffled tones when we hear someone has depression or anxiety or any other mental illness. It's not their fault. No, someone with anxiety or depression, an eating disorder, schizophrenia or another mental illness can't just 'snap out of it' . . . just like you can't snap out of asthma.

If you're struggling right now – maybe feeling like it's all pointless; maybe you just want to shut yourself out from the world because it feels so hard – please know that you're not alone and things will get better. It's not weak to speak to someone, it's incredibly strong. It takes a lot of courage to say: 'I shouldn't have to feel like this. I'm not OK.'

Let's not bury ourselves in our doonas, but rather practise asking for help. And let's not whisper about mental health or avoid the topic. If everything feels too hard, make an appointment with your doctor and set up a time to a speak to a mental health-care professional. You'd be happy to help a friend who's overwhelmed, so grant yourself the same kindness.

Set clear boundaries

FACT: Standing up for yourself is scary. How do I know this? Because whenever I decide to do or say something, not in line with the status quo – which is pretty much every day – I feel fear creep in. The fear of being disliked, judged, criticised, laughed at, left out, yelled at, you name it.

I used to believe, like so many humans, that being 'likeable' was the most desirable trait. I was a people-pleaser at my own expense.

I'd say yes to things I felt I should do, then feel exhausted and depleted afterwards – resenting my decision AND the person whom I thought asked too much of me.

Do you ever feel:
* like you do things because you should? 'If I don't do it, she won't like me.'
* scared of saying no? 'If I don't agree, he will think I'm boring.'
* afraid to stand up for yourself? 'If I ask them to stop commenting on my weight, they won't understand.'
* like you mirror the people around you, even if it feels wrong? 'Everyone else is saying yes, so I'd better say yes as well.'

The truth is, we all crave the freedom to be ourselves. To say what we really think, eat what we really want to eat, wear what we really want to wear, and openly share what we really believe. But we also want to feel loved and accepted.

Life has tricked us into believing we'll only be loved if we show up as the prettiest, happiest, thinnest version of ourselves, and push anything 'undesirable' deep down where no one can see it.

There are days when the fear of being disliked will be enough to keep you quiet so you go with the flow, even if it feels all wrong. But here's the thing: setting boundaries helps keep you healthy, with enough energy for yourself.

If you're constantly serving others – and doing what you think is expected of you instead of what you really want to be doing – you'll become depleted and low in energy. While setting clear, healthy boundaries is essential, so is accepting that it's OK if not everyone likes and agrees with you.

No matter what you do, what you look like, how much you weigh, what you wear or what you believe, there will always be someone who doesn't accept you. You can be the juiciest peach, and yet some people simply don't enjoy peaches.

Care enough about yourself to say no

People are going to ask too much from you. That you can't control. You can either get angry with them for asking too much of you (this method doesn't work: I've tried) OR you can get good at setting clear boundaries.

Here's my own example: about once a week I get an email asking me to work for free. I've agreed in the past, but these types of requests always drain my energy and leave me feeling resentful. Instead of getting angry at people for asking me to do unpaid hours, I realised that I was the boss of my boundaries. So now I use this phrase to guide me: if it's not a 'Hell yes!' then it's a 'No thanks'. In other words, if it doesn't light you up and excite you from the very start – if you have to think about it – then it's probably best to say no. People will always ask too much of you. It's up to you to enforce your own boundaries because no one else is going to do it for you.

It's OK to disappoint others

How much are you willing to sacrifice yourself so that someone else can avoid disappointment? How much someone thinks you should be doing is more about them than you. How someone else feels about your body is a reflection on their own sense of self, not a true representation of your worth or wellbeing.

I spoke with clinical psychologist Talya Rabinovitz, who has dedicated her career to helping people avoid overwhelm and constant stress. She says most people aren't disappointing enough people! If you stop striving for the perfect body, trying to do the right thing all the time, who would you be disappointing?

* your parents?
* yourself?
* your doctor?
* your partner?

In order to prioritise yourself, it's going to mean letting go of some things. And probably disappointing others who have become familiar with how much you give to their lives, or how you maintain their sense of what should be done. You may need to have some difficult conversations with a partner or parent or child. Chances are, if you stand up for yourself, not everyone will be happy about it. And that's OK.

You don't need to sacrifice yourself, your health, to avoid disappointing someone else. You don't need to sacrifice your health – by going on a weight-loss diet – to appear healthier to someone. Are you willing to choose yourself? Is your daily mental wellbeing not way more valuable than someone else's momentary disappointment?

Also, is this imagined disappointment? Sometimes it is. We feel anxiety that someone may be disappointed. They may not have expressed disappointment, but we are disappointed in our body and so we imagine they will be disappointed too. Or perhaps the disappointment is real. They've made comments in the past. That has deeply hurt. I experienced many years of being told my body was a disappointment. My failure to have the perfect body was embarrassing and a weakness.

At some point, I had to decide that my body and my mental health was far more important than trying to micromanage someone else's response to my shape. Those people critiquing your body, are they perfectly shaped? Are they free from cellulite and bumps and ingrown hairs?

Nobody has a perfect-looking body. So those people who are so disappointed in your body are really struggling with the shame they feel around their own body. Or the messages they have been given by literally everyone since they were born that if we aren't constantly striving to have a perfect body, we are failures. Their problems with their body are not yours.

We need to be OK with disappointing more people. The alternative is continuing to disappoint ourselves.

Being OK with not being liked

So many people I know end up being the passenger in their own life (as I used to be). But you – my dear – you are the main character in your life. You need to be in the driver's seat, and choose which direction you are going to go.

But to do this, you need strong healthy boundaries and the ability to say NO – even if it means being disliked. Accepting that being disliked is inevitable frees you up to choose what you REALLY want to do instead of living your life for other people. According to palliative care nurses, the most common regret of the dying is a wish they'd had the courage to live a life true to themselves, not the life others expected. Courage is a choice. Your choice. It takes courage to create change and challenge the status quo.

The beauty is when we have the courage to show up as our REAL selves, we also give the people around us permission to do the same. And it's a relief to those around us because now they can finally speak their mind too. Courage is contagious: give it to yourself and to others. Ready to feel the fear and do – or say or write or wear or sing or dance – it anyway?

Energy management review

✎ What do you spend your energy on?

Rank these life areas from 1 to 10 based on which you most often spend your energy on:

— Health

— House

— Career

— Family

— Friends

— Relationship

— Food

— Style

— Hobbies

— Sleep

Now repeat the exercise, this time ranking the life areas from 1 to 10 based on what is most important to you. Is there a mismatch between how you're currently spending your energy and what you would like to spend your energy on? Simply becoming aware of any mismatch is a really good first step.

✎ What sucks energy from you?

What opens more tabs in your mind? Write a list of the things that draw energy from you without refuelling you. For example:

* people who talk about themselves all the time
* compulsive shopping
* compulsive cleaning and reorganising
* having too much stuff
* drinking alcohol
* too many/too few social plans
* not enough 'me' time

How can you reduce or eliminate these energy-drainers from your life? Some things are, of course, unavoidable, like taxes. But sometimes, we fall into the trap of living a certain way without recognising that it's not serving us.

✎ What gives you energy?

What closes tabs and gives you more space for living? Add items that give you more energy. For example:

* going for a mental-health walk
* reading a magazine in a cafe
* music
* swimming in the ocean
* going on a holiday or minibreak
* meditating
* going to bed earlier
* speaking to a psychologist or friend
* drinking enough water/eating enough

Reducing the number of things that take energy away from you is important. But so is adding more of the things that light you up. From my own experience with burnout, adding more of these things helped me feel like I was living life again, rather than just churning through it. Adjusting this ratio so there are more energy-giving activities than energy-draining activities can help the chores and to-do lists feel a little more purposeful. There are downloadable worksheets for the activities in this book available at *lyndicohen.com/bookresources*

A Better Way To Be Healthy

Essential takeaways

* Rest and self-care can help to reduce your stress, helping you feel better in your body and yourself. This is why it's a core habit within the hierarchy.

* Rest isn't watching TV while writing to-do lists or scrolling on social media. Prioritise real rest, whatever that means for you.

* Practise being forgiving and kind to yourself. You don't have to love yourself. Being kind is the act; the result is loving yourself.

* We chase self-improvement because we don't feel good enough as we are. If we accepted ourselves a little more, perhaps we'd finally stop feeling like we're chasing an unattainable goal.

* Choose to forgive yourself for being imperfect. You may find more connection with others when you're willing to turn up as your perfectly flawed, human self.

* Make your own lunch first. Or at least at the same time as you cater to the needs of others. Fill up your water bottle, pack food for yourself and perhaps a warm jumper, too!

* Practise lowering your standards while simultaneously being OK with asking and receiving help.

* There is no shame in having a mental illness. Make an appointment with a psychologist or mental health-care professional.

* Accepting that being disliked is inevitable can free you up to choose what you REALLY want to do instead of living your life for other people.

Chapter 10.

The secret to habits that stick

If your all-or-nothing mindset means you're either
obsessively exercising at the gym every freakin' day
or barely moving your body, it's time for a new
(much more balanced) way of being. It's time to stop
counting macros or almonds and start counting
happy memories instead.

Health fact: Swap rice for cauliflower and you can lose 88 per cent of the joy you get from food. (I'm pro-cauliflower but you're allowed to eat rice as well.)

Note: Not an actual fact! Ha!

Bonus health fact: When it comes right down to it, health is about consistency, not chia seeds. Are you surprised?

Enjoyable movement

As we've discussed, one of the most important things when it comes to healthy living is the enjoyment factor. On Level 2 of the hierarchy of healthy habits is enjoyable movement, a core habit. This doesn't involve rigorous circuit sessions or sweating so much that you look like you've just been for a swim. Enjoyable movement is about active living, including more incidental but nice-to-do activity in your day, from walking your dog to going for a dip down at the local pool.

Examples of enjoyable movement:
* Stretching your body.
* Dancing to old-school Britney while you make dinner.
* Walking your dog.
* Going on a hike.
* Going down the slide with your kids at the playground.
* Mental-health walks.
* Window shopping and browsing, especially fun on a rainy day.
* Doing a chill yoga class.
* Riding your bikes to drop the kids off at school.
* Taking the stairs.

* Walking to the postbox like an eighteenth-century maiden.
* Going horseriding.
* Signing up to dance or acting class.
* Rollerblading.

The purpose of enjoyable movement isn't necessarily fitness (though that can be a side effect). Rather, it's about getting the feel-good benefits of moving your body around. Doing more movement can make you feel more joyful. More energetic, too. It can help you feel like you're taking part in life as you're getting outside more or trying new things.

Children are perfect exemplars of enjoyable movement. They don't think about exercise. They play, run up hills for no reason or try to touch their toes. They dance when music comes on, injecting more fun into their lives. The aim is to reclaim a bit of this, to move from being a witness to life to being more of a participant. You're partaking in active living and becoming a more energetic version of yourself.

We've talked about how eating kale leaves with activated almonds for a day isn't going to transform your health (and nor is it something you need to do to be healthy). True health is what happens when you do healthy habits consistently, not as a one-off. And to become as reliably consistent as the perpetual closing-down sale at the local rug store, healthy things can't feel like punishment, a chore or a bore.

A chore is how exercise and moving my body felt for me during the decade I was dieting. Back then, the sole reason I exercised was to lose weight, which meant I only did the types of exercise I'd read about that were 'best for weight loss', completely dismissing enjoyable movement options as a waste of time because they didn't burn enough calories. I joined a boot camp that made me feel like throwing up. I was constantly sore, battered or injured. I ran for kilometres each day, even though I loathed it, chafing the inside of my thighs red (and somehow my underarms too).

At one point (in the height of my eating-disorder days) I would force myself to run along a busy highway with polluted air, thinking it would motivate me to keep running; believing that the passing motorists who saw me thought, 'Look at that girl who can't run.' I imagined people were judging me and my body while I exercised, which felt like a barrier to exercising. Truth is that no one even noticed me sweating and stressing about my body. I had recruited self-loathing to propel me along the pavement, somehow believing that it would help me like myself more.

As a result, I detested exercising. It was deeply tied to the number on the scale. Moving my body felt like punishment for eating, something I HAD to do for fear of weight gain. So would you believe it when I tell you that I found it really hard to exercise consistently? Woah, what a shock. I bet you didn't see that coming. We all LOVE doing things that feel hard, gruelling, painful and punishing, right? Attaching health habits to weight loss is a dangerous business; it's a recipe for inconsistent, joyless living.

Ten years later, at my high school reunion, an old friend reminded me of this: clearly it was something I thought was 'healthy' motivation and worth sharing with others. Oh, the disorder.

Joy is fundamental to long-lasting health

When I quit dieting, I also quit doing intense exercise I hated, resigning from the gym membership I paid for without ever going and unsubscribing from all their annoying emails where weight-loss advice was dished out under the guise of wellbeing or self-care. During my recovery, there was a long time when I couldn't bring myself to move my body. It felt poisonous and tainted. And honestly? It was a relief to no longer have to force myself to do it.

Slowly, I began reintroducing enjoyable movement into my life. Key to this was not attaching weight-loss goals to my health goals and ensuring that everything I did felt joyful. At first, I started with enjoyable, slow walks. Listening to a podcast or new playlist was (and still is) an important part of it. Still, to this day, walking is my baseline form of movement.

Oh, and I got a good sports bra that wasn't too tight around my chest or pushing my boobs up into my chin. Hard to find!

I'd always considered stretching to be pointless as it didn't burn enough calories, but once I realised that there was real value in simply moving my body and doing things that made it feel good regardless of the calories it burned, my relationship with movement shifted.

As time went on, as I found moving my body became more enjoyable, I began to naturally crave more and different movement. So next I started doing yoga, something I wouldn't have considered 'proper' exercise before because it didn't make me sweat.

Mental health movement

Walking is non-negotiable for my mental health. My life is a million times (an exaggeration, but you get the point) better when I walk. You know those little things in life you need to do to feel like you're not drowning? Walking is mine. Let's backtrack: I started this year turning the microscope on my #mentalhealth. I tracked things like sleep, steps and hours spent on my phone. What came from that jumble of numbers was an undeniable link: when I walked more, I slept better and turned the dial down on my anxiety. Bye, insomnia. Hello, more energy.

You see, on the days I walked, my body was tired, as was my brain. Rather than waiting until my head hit the pillow to run things over a tonne of times, my brain had already had time for the Big Think while I was out walking. So when those feelings of pointlessness knock at my head, I know I need to lace up my shoes, even if I don't want to, or I feel I don't have time. Just because I don't ALWAYS feel like going for a walk doesn't mean it's unenjoyable. Some days it's just not as flow-y. Everyone needs a place for some pent-up anxiety to exit. Mine happens with each footstep that hits the pavement.

✎ Find enjoyable movement

Ask yourself:

* How did I enjoy moving my body when I was a child? Did I love playing sports or dancing? This question offers precious insights into what you actually enjoy, before your weight and how you look were part of the equation.
* How would I exercise for fun if it had no impact on my weight?

A note about fitness watches

I really like having a watch that counts how many steps I've done, lets me know if I'm getting enough quality sleep or alerts me when I'm a bit too stressed. It's a mental-health tool and it serves me well. But I'm at the point where, if I'm having a lousy day, if I notice that I've barely shuffled beyond my desk, I can gently remind myself that a walk will probably help me feel better without any guilt.

And when I don't hit my steps target, I don't beat myself up for it. I don't jump around in the bathroom while brushing my teeth or skip around my apartment just to get a green tick of validation before bed (I used to be that person during my decade of dieting). I'm now blissfully unattached to the number I get each day, using it solely for research and self-care purposes.

If you feel guilty when you don't get enough steps, if it feels like yet another rule, then perhaps a fitness watch is fuelling an unhealthy relationship with movement. It might be time to pop your watch into your bedside drawer until a later date. Or sell it. Either way, I do strongly recommend that you turn off how many calories you've supposedly burned that day (unless you're an athlete with a healthy relationship with food and you need to eat more to fuel your workouts).

The enjoyment zone

Here's the thing. Twenty minutes of exercise you enjoy is ALWAYS better than an hour at the gym that never happens because you hate going. The healthiest exercise truly is the exercise you enjoy the most, not the exercise that burns the most calories.

But what's the point or benefit of going softly, gently and enjoyably along? Well, small habits done consistently add up to something big and wonderful. And the key to being consistent is enjoyment. Because when you enjoy what you're doing, you'll likely find it so much easier to be consistent. Without the struggle. No willpower needed. Instead of feeling like going to the gym is something you 'should' do, you look forward to moving your body because it's something that lights you up. So if that means you choose to go for a walk instead of a run (because you loathe running but don't mind the idea of going for a stroll around a park while listening to an audiobook) then that's fab. You may start going to salsa or swing dance classes because it's enjoyable. Or choose to sign up to a sports team, socialising and moving your body while having fun. Because you enjoy it, you'll find you naturally do it more consistently, and that's a real prize.

The same applies to healthy eating.[1] If it feels like a punishment, you're doing it wrong. I don't know about you, but dieting kinda ruined my ability to see healthy food as something desirable. Dieting advice told me to strip out anything unnecessary or too high in calories. What I was left with was dull, boring and bland-tasting healthy food; hardly something I could look forward to or view positively. When you remove all the fun, enjoyable ingredients from healthy food you change your very perception.

There is so much benefit in making healthy food enjoyable and something you actually get excited about. Instead of forcing yourself to ingest steamed broccoli and chicken, you lap up food with flavour, along with all the nutrients.

If you want to be more consistent, and you want to have more joy in your life, and like yourself more, then let's forget the 'fat burn' zone. Or the 'heart rate' zone. The most important place to be in is in the enjoyment zone. Something that can apply to exercise, healthy eating and many other areas of your life.

Swap it

* Stop doing high-intensity workouts that you hate and choose enjoyable movement.
* Stop avoiding carbs, because they are your body's preferred source of energy.
* Stop quitting sugar, because making foods 'off-limits' only makes you crave them more.
* Stop counting calories and recording everything you eat in an app, because it's depressing, unsustainable and sure as hell won't measure your worth.

Cooking more at home

Cooking at home more sits on Level 2 of the hierarchy of healthy habits because it can make a big difference to your wellbeing. Research by Johns Hopkins Bloomberg School of Public Health in 2014 found that people who cook more at home are healthier.[2] Oh, and you bet they also save money. Of course, if you're working crazy hours, it's going to be a whole lot trickier to cook at home, and research confirms that people who work 35 hours a week or more tend to cook less.[3]

But the research that I find most interesting is this: in general, people who cooked five or more times a week at home ate healthier meals. They consumed less sugar, fewer carbs and less fat than those who didn't cook as much. Simply cooking more at home, even if it's not 'perfectly' healthy food, is almost always going to be good news for your health.

This may be because, when compared with fast food options, it's almost always healthier to eat at home. You may be more likely to cook with vegetables, and use healthier cooking methods like baking or grilling rather than deep-frying. Even if your style of eating out involves trying to choose a healthier option, generally (and it does depend on what you cook at home), you may still not be getting as nutritious a dish as if you were at home, cooking a wholesome meal.

Possible new habit: Aim to cook at home one more night a week

How many nights a week do you usually cook at home? Do you find you're spending a large amount of money eating out? Even cooking at home one extra night a week can be helpful, especially if you double the recipe so you have another home-cooked meal for the next day (this then counts as two home-cooked meals)!

Investing a bit of time to improve your cooking skills is a smart thing to do. Rather than spending $60 a week on expensive supplements, sign up for a cooking class and learn skills that will last you a lifetime. You will end up saving a tonne of money in the long term, will likely eat healthier and won't have to struggle to eat any average-tasting food you prepared.

Ditch tasteless, diet food for enjoyable options

Dieting ruined salads for me. Magazines articles 'warning' us of the hidden calories in salad dressing. Advice to ask for dressing on the side. The myth that there are 'fattening' or 'bad' salads. And it's left us with pathetic bowls of

And I can never look at jelly in quite the same way!

wilted lettuce leaves that are depressing to anyone with taste buds. It also left us with the outdated thinking that pleasure is associated with unhealthy food and not with healthy food.

I enjoy food too much to waste time eating boring salads. The only reason I eat salads is because of the tasty dressing. Yes, I get it. Salad dressings contain calories, sugar and fat. And yes, cafés can sometimes add lots of salad dressing (too much for some people's preferences).

But here's the thing. If adding some delicious salad dressing helps you happily devour countless vegetables, it's a major nutrition win. And damn tasty, too!

Honestly? Most people don't eat enough salad. And you know what makes you want to eat a salad? Salad dressing. And the extra yummy bits on top that excite you like avocado or nuts or feta (because feta makes everything beta).

Not only are salads palatable with salad dressing but – fun fact – adding salad dressing helps you absorb fat-soluble nutrients (vitamins A, D, E and K). With salad dressing, it's likely that you'll also stay fuller for longer because fat can also help make you feel satisfied after eating.

You deserve to enjoy food AND you deserve to be healthy. The two are NOT mutually exclusive. I say, if a bit of salad dressing helps you get through a whole plate of the healthy stuff, then drizzle away.

A lovely follower of mine, named May, got it. 'I bought a bag of salad this week that came with a serving of dressing in a little bag as that was the only packed salad they had. I put the dressing over the salad. I would have NEVER EVER eaten store-bought or "unclean" dressing normally, but I didn't even think. I ate it. I was happy. I'm so much more relaxed around food now.'

Hooray for May! And hooray for you, and this new permission you have to actually enjoy healthy food. It's revolutionary I know, but I say we should bring back abundant salads. Loaded, luscious, I-can't-wait-to-eat-it salads.

Make abundant salads that don't taste crap

Leaves are a good place to start. But don't be stingy with the carbs, either: include wholegrains, like brown rice or quinoa. Add pasta, like orzo or couscous or spirals. How fun! You can have a salad with just leaves as the base, just carbs or a mix of both. Forget the rules about how to balance the plate according to portion size. Balance it to your appetite! Personally, I like a mix of it all, depending on whether the moon is in the seventh house.

Once your base is sorted, rummage through the kitchen for all sorts of things. Yes, add colourful vegies (I'm a big fan of those precut coleslaw salad mixtures: easy to add to a bowl in a jiffy). When your plate is loaded with vegies, bring in the tasty stuff, and don't be shy. Avocado, feta and delicious dressing. Don't forget some crunchy, crispy bits: toasted seeds, those curly, crispy noodle things or corn chips. Yes, you heard me! Add chips to a salad. Do what it takes to eat more vegetables and if that means adding some chips, I'm all for it.

My client Melody had a salad-induced light-bulb moment. She said, 'This is liberating for me. I enjoy making salad dressings and have also allowed myself to buy a roast chicken or two (and it turns out there's an amazing roast chicken shop on my way home from work that I've always kept off limits, but now I love adding it to my salads).' Smart thinking, Melody. You're my kinda lady.

A packet of coleslaw mixture combined with roast chicken is dinner done. Add the dressing from the packet and those crispy bits. Doesn't have to get fancier than that, but you might just find adding some avocado or a tin of drained chickpeas will surprise and delight. That's what this is about.

How can you make healthy food taste truly delectable? What would transform it from a compromise to feeling like first prize?

Make vegies suck less

If you hate vegetables and salads, chances are that you've got the cooking skills of a toddler OR you simply haven't yet been informed that it's OK and a very clever thing to make vegetables taste insanely good. Consider this your permission slip. And while you're with me, here are some ideas on how to make that happen.

* Sprinkle cheese, such as parmesan or cheddar, on your vegies.
* Add panko breadcrumbs, and your favourite herbs and spices.

Not actually. How lush my salad is depends on my hunger levels. I like science too much to fluff about with the meaning of constellations but if it's your spiritual jam, go for it.

* Splash on extra virgin olive oil for healthy fats and yumminess.
* Ditch boiling as a cooking method and try baking, stir-frying or airfrying for better browning (and thus better taste).

Remember: in my world no vegetables are off limits, even the carb-y ones that contain 'points'. Boiled, baked or mashed potato is not a treat food. Swap perfect eating for enjoyable eating. You'll find a pot of consistency at the end of that rainbow. When we start demonising perfectly healthy, nutritious foods like vegetables, when we believe that only perfect and 'clean' ingredients are permitted, we make food more overwhelming and it probably makes us less likely to get our recommended five or more serves a day. If adding some yummy cheese or crunchy bits means you actually hit your daily veggie targets, you'll be winning.

Creating a healthy home environment

Your environment has a pretty huge impact on how you eat. Just think about how differently you eat when you're on holiday. When on holiday, you have totally different food cues. So what is a food cue? It's something that makes you think about food or eating. It might be a place, a specific shelf, a time of day or something you see. Ever seen a commercial for fried chicken and then really wanted some? Have you suddenly had an urge for chocolate only after spotting it sitting on a shelf in the pantry? Food cues are everywhere. And if you've been a dieter, you might even be more sensitive to them than non-dieters.

Some more examples of food cues:
* In the grocery store where checkouts are lined with chocolates, lollies and mints. It's a little reminder to stock up on these impulse purchases, and supermarkets place these items right in a spot where you'll be hanging about before you purchase. Smart for them, tricky for us.
* Another food cue might be a time of a day, like school pickup or the drive home from work. If you often have something to eat around that time, hopping in the car or public transport might just be enough to trigger a thought about eating, and it may create specific cravings for you too.

While there are plenty of food cues we can't control, there are a bunch we can have some influence over, without making us feel deprived.

Modify your pantry

You're allowed to eat anything you want, whenever you want. This is important to remember so that you don't trigger more out-of-control eating. But I'm also an advocate for building a healthy food environment for yourself. Why? Well, we tend to eat what's around us. At the end of the day, I want to eat yummy foods, especially when I'm stressed or tired or all of the above. With a tiny dictator (ahem, I mean toddler), this is inevitable. So, building a healthy food environment really does help.

This is not about creating a perfect healthy home. We want to aim for a 'healthy enough' environment, avoiding the temptation to turn your pantry into a perfect eater's sanctuary where only hemp seeds and raw unsalted almonds may hang out. You've got to find the balance that works for you so that you don't feel deprived (very important so we don't trigger more emotional eating or increased cravings from feeling restricted). But at the same time, you're trying to create an environment that supports you to be healthy.

Back in my dieting years, I'd eat perfectly when I was out in public so others could see how committed I was to weighing less, only to end up eating all the foods at home in private. Nowadays, I've given myself permission to do the exact opposite. This means I eat my favourite foods when I'm out: for example, ordering a flaky croissant with my morning coffee. Having ice cream after a delicious dinner out. And my home environment is built to help me eat healthier. Sure, I have things like a block of chocolate, biscuits and some popcorn in my house, but they don't dominate the pantry. They are there when I want them, but because I have permission to eat them anytime, I don't feel the need to load my kitchen with them anymore. Generally I find it's easier for me to eat healthily when my environment is supporting my choices.

That said, you might feel differently. It's important to feel that nothing is off limits. If the idea of not having certain foods in your house makes you feel like they are forbidden, if it feels more like a sentence rather than a choice, then you've got to do you. The aim is to create an environment that supports you to be healthy, and that may mean five different types of ice cream in your freezer or it might not.

Try online grocery shopping

Food companies and supermarkets want to sell their products to you. Their job is to make food as appealing as possible. If you find that you often come back from the store with a bunch of items you didn't really intend to buy, try online grocery shopping. It's become quite a streamlined, easy process these days, and it may help save you time and money. Once you've set it up, it's easy to reorder items and set up recurring deliveries.

If you genuinely enjoy grocery shopping, there's no need to overhaul something that's working for you.

Reorganise your fridge

If you're like me and forget about the product that's in the crisper, only remembering about it once it's sad or mouldy, try reorganising your fridge. Place your fresh produce on the main shelves, especially fruit so that it's easy to find. This means that meats and proteins and rarely used condiments can actually go into the crisper. No need for them to be taking up precious food cue real estate! The benefit of having your fruit and other produce in clear line of sight is that you might find you're more likely to eat them.

Essential takeaways

* Enjoyable movement isn't punishing or gruelling. It's about active living, finding fun and joyful ways to move your wonderful body.

* Moving your body may be key for your mental health, allowing time for the big think. There are many benefits, including better mental health, more consistency and thus more energy, when you stop thinking exercise and movement is about burning calories.

* Cooking at home more is a core habit. And it doesn't need to be done perfectly either. People who cook at home tend to eat healthier (and save money) so maybe try doing it one or three more nights a week.

* Make abundant, great-tasting salads instead of sad boring bowls. Healthy food shouldn't feel like a compromise. Ditch the idea that all food must be 'clean' or perfect. If adding more enjoyable ingredients, with some added calories, means you eat healthier, it's a major win.

* Create a healthy home environment that supports you. You might change the types of foods you buy for your home and give yourself permission to eat ice cream when out with friends as opposed to secretly eating it at home because it feels shameful to do in public. Try online shopping or reorganising your fridge.

Chapter 11.

Enrichment habits

Now, it's time to add enrichment habits (Level 3), which do exactly what they say they will on the box. Once you've got a solid base of health with your basic needs met and your core habits fulfilled, you may choose to add enrichment habits: things like mindful eating, fitness, crowding and including a variety of foods add an additional layer of goodness into your life.

A new approach to fitness

I love exercise and movement – whatever you like to call it. But I'm not a fan of fitness. Well, not the version of fitness you see these days: the fitness in the magazines I bought when I was a teen, with sculpted bodies and visible abs. I'm not a fan of what fitness has come to mean.

* Gym-mirror selfies to prove to others we exercised.
* Abs one day, legs and glutes the next, repeat every day until you die.
* Before-and-after photos in crop tops or bikinis.
* 12-week body challenges.
* Eating the same foods on repeat, because it's 'safe'.
* Chasing unhealthy body-fat percentages.
* Powdered protein supplements in place of actual meals.
* Weird 'energy' drinks, some containing illicit substances.

This fitness culture isn't representing health. Fitness has come to be about looking a certain way, whereas health is about feeling a certain way.

Fitness culture often encourages you to:
* obsess about food
* track progress by how your body looks rather than how it feels
* consistently undereat
* dehydrate yourself to get more definition
* eat foods on repeat (not amazing for gut health and immunity)
* use diet supplements, placing an extra load on your liver
* eat a tonne of sugar right before a fitness competition

It's time to move away from this aesthetic-obsessed fitness culture and move towards real fitness.

Real fitness is one of the enrichment habits in the hierarchy of healthy habits. But it's about building a healthier heart through getting your heart rate up, without sacrificing other parts of your life, including your social life. Health-centered fitness is about setting realistic goals and choosing exercises you enjoy, irrespective of how many calories they burn. You can lift weights or go running. Join a volleyball team or swim or run an ultramarathon. Or start with a sweaty, fun dance class.

If enjoyable movement is the starting point, then fitness is levelling up. We know that moving your body, getting your heart pumping, doing resistance training and impact workouts are brilliant things for your body. Diet culture has scared us away from reaping the benefits of fitness, because we've come to associate deprivation and punishment with more intense forms of movement.

What if you could find a form of fitness that you did because you enjoyed how it made you feel? Because you liked the version of yourself when you do things like go for a run or lift heavy things? Can we untether fitness from the grips of diet culture so that we can get the mood-boosting, life-extending, energy-enhancing benefits of engaging in fitness?

Is your exercise routine working for you?

Without gym selfies or before-and-after photos, how can you actually tell if your exercise or movement habits are working for you? Here are some non-appearance-related metrics to take a squiz at.

* It's easy to be consistent.
* You crave or miss exercise when you don't get a chance to do it.
* You feel stronger and more agile.
* You're able to listen to your body and adjust intensity depending on your energy levels or how your muscles feel.
* You've got more energy when you exercise.
* You feel better in your body.
* You sleep better at night.
* Your mood is lifted after a good workout. At minimum, it isn't worse.
* You almost always feel better after you've exercised.
* Exercise doesn't feel like a chore, but rather something you get to do.

Intuitive exercise

Here's a little idea that's kinda the opposite of what the fitness world tells us. Intuitive exercise isn't about looking good, it's about listening to your lovely, smart body to help you feel good. Simply put, it's about adjusting how you move your body based on how you feel and how you want to feel.

Don't be fooled. Intuitive exercise isn't about giving up. You can be an athlete and be an intuitive exerciser. In fact, it's a brilliant way to get more joy from exercise, avoid burnout and boredom and sidestep injuries because you respond to the first clues your body gives you that something doesn't feel right.

Intuitive exercise is about respecting your limits, avoiding comparison and exercising to feel good.

Here's what intuitive exercise looks like:

* Giving yourself permission to do a gentle workout instead of a high-intensity one.
* Noticing niggles in your body and easing up when you get a little nudge that something isn't feeling 100 per cent right. This helps you avoid getting injured.
* Taking rest days when you need them.
* Ramping up workouts for more of a challenge on days when you have more energy and it feels right in your body to do so.
* Doing movement that your body enjoys instead of committing to something that you hate doing, just because you think you 'should' do it or someone else is posting about their workout.
* Noticing how the exercise habits of others impact on your sense of self.
* Embracing feel-good movement, instead of exercising because you're trying to look good or get a certain aesthetic.
* Movement that feels enjoyable and fun.

Sometimes, while I was on one of my mental-health walks, I'd start jogging. Naturally, because I felt energetic, and because I wanted to. Oh, how lovely. And with time, I naturally found myself coming back to high-intensity stuff because it sounded fun. I got into lifting weights, loving the focus on functionality over appearance.

How do you know if you're exercising too much?

Too much or too little? It's a tricky balance to find. It's a situation where we can apply the Goldilocks principle so that you're not depleting your body further by trying to do too much. Here's a guide that may be able to help you know if you're over- or underexercising.

Underexercising	Healthy exercise	Overexercising
✶ Generally, you may feel low in energy and tired all the time.*	✶ Often feel energised during the day.	✶ Feel sore all the time.
✶ Energy may reduce as the day progresses.*	✶ Experience more energy after exercising.	✶ Feel depleted and exhausted after exercising.
✶ May have trouble sleeping if you don't use energy during the day.*	✶ Motivated to do it because you enjoy it and like how you feel afterwards.	✶ Driven by guilt or rules about how much you 'should' be exercising; you'd like to do less but feel you can't.
✶ You may have normal menstrual cycles.	✶ May still have normal menstrual cycles.	✶ Your periods may stop; can contribute to lower iron levels.
✶ You never have enough time to get to the gym.	✶ You make time for your favourite form of exercise.	✶ Miss out on life because your workout is more important than other plans with friends.
✶ You may not need as much food to fulfil your body's energy needs.	✶ May find your appetite increases to match your energy output.	✶ If you eat more than planned, you feel you need to exercise more.

* These symptoms may also be caused by something else. If you feel exhausted all the time, make an appointment with your GP to try to get to the root cause.

If you feel like you might be exercising too much, then your doctor is a good person to speak to first. You could ask to get a blood test done, and ask to speak to a psychologist.

Note: some of you divine humans might already love high-intensity workouts. That's brilliant. I'm not poo-pooing high-intensity exercise (though it can make you want to do poo-poo). The key message is that you should do whatever movement is enjoyable for you, high or low, slow or fast. As you were. Hakuna matata. Keep enjoying!

✎ Make it enjoyable

If fitness is something you're ready to work on within your hierarchy of healthy habits, how can you turn it into something enjoyable? What fitness goal would you like to achieve that is disconnected from burning calories or looking a certain way?

Mindful eating

Mindful eating is paying attention to the food you eat. It's about eating in the present moment, generally while you're sitting at a table. It's about savouring the taste, texture, temperature and smell of your food. And it's about being aware of how hungry you are before, during and after your meal. Why does this even matter? Why is it classed as an enrichment habit, something worth investing in?

When we don't eat mindfully, we may be more likely to overeat. We may eat quickly, not enjoying our food as much as we can. It is near impossible to be a mindful eater when you're yet to tick off other more important habits on the hierarchy. If your body doesn't trust that it's going to get enough food, it can drive you into a state of fearing that the food will run out or may be taken away. This is a huge barrier to slowing down and being present with your meal.

This is why we must first address the basic need of eating enough food, located in prime position on Level 1 in the hierarchy of healthy habits. From there, building intuitive eating into our habit stack can help you tune into your body's energy needs, and listen for important cues. After that, you may find mindful eating a lot easier to achieve.

Eating mindfully is a seriously important step to tackling your complicated relationship with food. Because when you eat mindfully, you have time to notice your hunger and the emotions you have around food. You can finally experience the food in front of you. And you're likely to feel more connected to and more comfortable in your body, because you're actually listening to what it needs.

Why don't we eat mindfully?

This crazy, lightning-fast culture we live in has banished the traditional mealtime etiquette our grandparents valued. Banished it so far back, it's buried deep in the storage room that has become the boot of your car. My grandmother certainly did not eat in front of the TV, at least not most of the time. I clearly remember her politely asking us to sit up straight, return our utensils to our plates between bites, and keep our elbows off the table (which, in hindsight, actually meant that we were naturally forced to eat more mindfully. Mind blown over here).

So, why have we lost touch with how to eat?

1. **You think you have no time.** Have you ever taken a bite of food and immediately started loading up your fork before you had a chance to even taste the food? The next time this happens, ask yourself, 'Why am I rushing?' The food isn't going to run out. If you genuinely have five minutes to eat your sandwich between back-to-back meetings, you're forgiven. A human's gotta eat. But if you have at least 10 to 20 minutes to eat, you probably have enough time to enjoy your meal and slow down a little.

2. **You restrict yourself or aren't eating enough.** As you now know, restricting yourself doesn't just refer to a physical restriction, like avoiding carbs, banning chocolate or following a strict diet like paleo or keto. Just because you're not 'on a diet' doesn't mean you're not restricting yourself. Emotional and physical hunger not only make you feel guilty about the food you ate, but they also make it really difficult to enjoy and be mindful about how you're eating it. Check to make sure you are eating enough food.

3.   **You don't want to waste food.** There's something very human about wanting to finish everything on your plate. Perhaps it's something you grew up hearing as a child? But there's a BIG difference between wasting food and simply having leftovers. I hate food waste but valuing your body's energy needs is also important stuff. My tip? If you aren't hungry, don't pressure yourself to eat. Store whatever's left over in the fridge for later or in the freezer (if appropriate) for an easy meal in a few weeks' time. Hurray for leftovers.

Eating more mindfully

Modern life makes eating mindfully a real challenge. Here are a few simple practices that will help you stay in the present moment and, hopefully, start to really enjoy and savour the act of eating.

1. Put down your phone

If you choose one thing from this list, start here. Eating without a screen in front of you will automatically shift your awareness to the food. Eating with a screen in front of you makes it virtually impossible to do so. Imagine you're at the cinema with a giant box of popcorn in your lap. It's too easy to polish off the entire box! The excitement unfolding on our screens – from the never-ending social media feed to Ryan Gosling's latest romcom – is too stimulating and numbs all other sensations. Yep, that includes the taste of your food, the texture of the food, and how satiated you feel during your meal.

When you're tuned into your favourite TV show, it's hard to be tuned into your body's innate cues. When we eat in front of the TV, we can condition our brains to crave food when we flick on a show. This might be another reason to help explain those niggly, out-of-nowhere food desires you have after dinner, while sitting on the couch and your new TV series. Aiming to sit at the table to eat can be a simple, enjoyable habit. For parents, it's a brilliant way to model healthy habits and teach your kids to eat mindfully, too.

Possible new habit: try to eat most of your main meals sitting at the table, and keep devices out of sight.

An open letter to nutrition and fitness professionals from Lyndi Cohen

Your job is to make people the healthiest version of themselves, not the thinnest. Your clients and patients will come to you desperate to be made thinner, imagining that their lives will be infinitely better if they just weigh less. At times like this, remember: it's not your job to make people the thinnest version of themselves. You can do SO much more for them.

Hear them (with bucketloads of empathy) when they tell you how they hate their soft tummy that's never quite flat, or how they've spent years trying to weigh less. Then when they're ready, gently explain the beautiful, awesome truth that is: Their body has their back! And if they simply redirect their energy away from focusing on their weight – and put that glorious energy into adopting truly healthy habits bit by bit – their bodies will naturally find their sweet spots.

Remind them their bodies want them to be healthy. It's going to be different for everyone and something the BMI can't determine. Remind them that real health takes time. And let them know that it's time to finally stop fighting their bodies and, instead, learn to sit back and listen.

Not all people who diet will have an eating disorder but almost everyone who gets an eating disorder starts with a diet. Here's an idea. It's not OK to give a larger person advice on how to lose weight if we wouldn't give that same advice to someone with an eating disorder, otherwise, aren't we just giving people eating-disorder advice? Most people with eating disorders go unnoticed, undiagnosed and untreated because they don't look like they have an eating disorder.

Give your clients permission to know it's time to stop recording everything they eat in apps (as though it can measure their worth when it sure as hell can't). Tell them it's OK – and beneficial – to stop counting macros and cutting out whole food groups.

Don't make them take before photos for an upcoming 12-week challenge and pretend it's for their wellbeing. Do not assume they are signing up to the gym to lose weight. And please don't encourage them to finish a workout by saying, 'Now you can feel less guilty about what you ate on the weekend.'

Whatever you do, help them (one healthy habit at a time) become the healthiest, best, happiest versions of themselves. THIS is the real work that you're here to do.

2. Start a tradition

This is probably my favourite tip. It's also the most fun and a great one if you have kids. Pick a meal – any meal will do, but preferably one where everyone is home. Dinner is an obvious choice, but it could be breakfast for some families. Sit down and eat together. Ask everyone to share something they are grateful for or learned that day. If you're not getting any traction, feel free to comment on the weather. You can extend this time into the kitchen by cooking as a family. Consider investing in a learning tower (a convertible booster/stepstool) or buy some child-friendly knives so they can help with simple tasks like chopping lettuce. Or ask them to mix granola with their hands!

3. Slow down

Perhaps you're worried there won't be enough: after years of dieting, it's common to hold a subconscious belief that food is not freely available, also known as 'food scarcity'. This can mean you eat very quickly – as if someone could take the food away at any moment. Addressing this fear, by first ensuring you are eating enough and breaking up with diet rules, is important. Because as long as you are on a diet or trying to be good, can you ever truly be a mindful eater?

I'm not asking you to emulate a camel and chew your food umpteen times. Honestly, I've tried it and it's just awkward. Especially if you're eating sweet potato mash. I do, however, encourage you to put down your fork or food while you're chewing, and not to pick it up again until you've swallowed that bite of food.

4. Eat when you're hungry

Practise intuitive eating (see Chapter 8). Tune in to your body and take a moment to see how you're feeling before eating. While you're eating, you can also check in with your body to see how eating more food is changing the way your body feels. Removing hunger? Helping me feel relaxed? What can you notice happening in your body?

5. Notice guilt

It's really challenging to eat mindfully when you're feeling guilty about what you're eating. It's like when you're having ice cream on waffles but you spend the entire time thinking about how many calories it has, how badly you want another waffle but don't want to be seen as greedy, or how much you're going to need to make up for it tomorrow. Guilt is the thief of joy when it comes to food. The antidote to guilt is to be present and mindful with your food (and to banish those faulty diet rules). When you notice those thoughts, remind yourself that you have full permission to eat that food. And you deserve to enjoy it. Focus your attention on the taste. Are the waffles crispy and buttery? How does the warm and cold sensation feel in your mouth? Letting yourself enjoy food can help you get more satisfaction from food. So see if you can choose to be a more mindful eater.

Crowding and variety

Old-school nutrition advice involved being handed a long list of food you weren't allowed to eat. New-school advice helps us eat more of the healthy stuff. Crowding and variety is the difference between positive and negative nutrition, and it's key to developing a healthy relationship with food. This can help explain why it's an enrichment habit, on Level 3 of the hierarchy of healthy habits.

What is crowding? Well, it's the opposite of restriction. And it works. Instead of focusing on what you're not allowed to eat, focus on what you want to eat more of. Naturally, you'll crowd out the less healthy options by filling up on the stuff that makes you feel good. This means you sidestep those intense cravings for foods you 'can't' have, you never feel like you're missing out and you're doing more of the healthy things that make you feel good.

My client Maggie had an anti-diet epiphany along these lines. 'It's taken me two years but I'm finally understanding this. Diets have you believe that you are living wrong and you must remove things from your life. REALITY is you need to ADD MORE: more vegies, more home-cooked meals, move more, sleep more, etc. It's taken two years for my mindset to really shift – and I know I'm not completely there – but I have to say it's a great feeling. Every time I dieted I would cry because I was hungry and I would also think, "How can I sustain this for life?" I'll never feel that way again, and I'm so glad!'

Maggie gets it. What if we redirected the energy we put into cutting out foods into adding more nutritious, tasty options into our diets? Like Maggie, what other habits can you crowd in beyond just food? More self-care, rest or clothing that fits? When it comes to food, there are lots of things you can crowd with.

Aim to eat:

* ✱ an extra serve of vegetables a day, working toward 5+ serves a day
* ✱ one to two pieces of a fruit a day, depending on what is in season
* ✱ legumes a few times a week
* ✱ wholegrains at least once a day, such as oats or brown rice
* ✱ nuts as a part of your diet, as a snack or in muesli or a smoothie

Only five per cent of Australians eat enough vegetables and half of us don't get enough fruit, yet we're constantly searching for the big secret when it comes to health. But as I've been telling you, I've got the secret! It's about adding more of the healthy stuff, not demonising less healthy stuff – and from there we can shift the balance to more nutrients.

Legumes are often forgotten, even though they're a brilliant source of fibre and plant-based protein and really affordable too. Maybe our obsession with trying to eat enough protein is distracting us from our real need to amp up how many vegetables we get in a day?

In fact, research from Blue Zones around the world shows that the one food eaten by people from all seven Blue Zones, from Japan to Greece, is legumes.[1] Soy beans, black beans, fava beans – all the beans – chickpeas, lentils and pulses. They somehow don't get nearly enough attention because we're too bedazzled by so-called 'superfoods' (which really is a marketing term rather than a nutrition concept). Adding more legumes to your diet can help you stretch your grocery bill further, eat less meat, eat more fibre (your gut health will be most grateful) and get more plant protein.

Blue Zones are places that have a high number of people who live to be over 100, living long and high-quality lives.

Like legumes, wholegrains are another often-forgotten food, and they've been hit hard by diet culture's insistence that we give up carbs. What if you didn't waste precious energy trying to eat less sugar or fat or whatever, but rather put that impressive intelligence towards eating more of the stuff that will help you live a longer and better life?[2]

Which are the healthiest fruits and vegetables, legumes or wholegrains to eat? The 'best' nut? Truthfully? The most benefit will come to those who constantly vary their diets, aiming for variety rather than perfection. People who eat the most diversity of plants in a week have the healthiest gut microbiota, crucial for immunity, healthy hormones and balanced moods.[3] Eating seasonally is a doable way to naturally vary what you eat – and snag the best deals on produce – ensuring your diet is loaded with variety.

The 'fruit is fattening' myth

Just so it's crystal clear. No, fruit isn't fattening. It's a brilliant food group to choose from every day, aiming for one to two serves a day. Why not more? Well, if you eat loads more fruit, you might not fit in all the other nutrients from important food groups. It's not about fruit being 'bad' for you. It's that variety is key. And if you do end up eating more fruit than you planned, and your tummy is fine with it and you feel good, it's really not something to beat yourself up over.

Even if what you're eating is really healthy, if you eat the same thing every day, it's not ideal. It's not as good for your gut microbiota (and health in general) as a diet loaded with diversity.

Aim to eat 30+ different types of plant-based foods a week to best support your gut health. Variety and crowding will help!

At the same time, you can't let crowding or 'eat more vegies' become yet another food rule. Tricky, I know, but I do believe it can be done. I've heard from clients who've felt guilty when they haven't included enough fruits and vegetables, giving them just one more thing to beat up on themselves about. Can we aim to crowd in more vegetables and fruit and then be compassionate, gentle and understanding when that doesn't happen?

Possible new habit: focus on one food to crowd in to your diet. Aim to hit the recommended intake for fruit (one to two serves a day) or crowd in an extra serve of vegies.

A Better Way To Be Healthy

Why I don't believe in 'cheat days'

The idea of a cheat day is rooted in diet culture. If your lifestyle is so hectic you need to periodically take breaks from it and cheat, then it's a sign that you're restricting and punishing yourself with far too many diet rules. Having cheat days sets you up for feeling guilty if you eat more or exercise less on non-cheat days. And it also encourages an all-or-nothing mindset, reinforcing large pendulum swings in your wellbeing. Food is always allowed. You don't need to wait for a cheat day.

Essential takeaways

* You can build strength or power, flexibility or stamina without buying into the disordered fitness culture BS.

* Exercise should give you more energy and feel good in your body. Intuitive movement is about listening and responding to your body, amping up or pulling back to respond in real time.

* Health-centered fitness is about setting realistic goals and choosing exercises that you enjoy, irrespective of how many calories they burn.

* Modern life plus diet rules makes eating mindfully a real challenge. Key to changing this is ensuring you're eating enough food, so that food doesn't feel like it has to be eaten in a hurry for fear of missing out.

* To practise eating mindfully, pop your phone down, sit at the table and try to tune in to the meal you're eating.

* Old-school nutrition advice involved being handed a long list of food you weren't allowed to eat. New-school advice helps us eat more of the healthy stuff.

* Fruit isn't fattening. Legumes are fabulous, so are wholegrains. Nuts and seeds, and things like loads of colourful vegies, spices and herbs, and tofu or tempeh can help contribute to getting 30+ different plant-based foods a week. Variety really is key to looking after your gut.

* Crowding in more of the healthy stuff – focusing on MORE rather than LESS – is the positive approach to nutrition that can shift your mindset, without getting caught up in diet nonsense.

Chapter 12.

Creating your ideal habits

The top level of the hierarchy of healthy habits is reserved for your ideal habits. These are the fabulous and fun things that enhance your life even further. It's not about ticking off something necessary for survival, but it's about finding your mojo.

Your ideal habits

They say you should fill up your cup and only let others drink from the overspill that lands in the saucer. Well, if the bottom three levels of the hierarchy pyramid are about filling up your cup, then your ideal habits are what can cause it to spill over.

For me, once I'm fulfilling all the lower levels of the hierarchy of healthy habits, then I can turn my attention to my ideal habits. Like vegetable gardening, something that lights me up. It helps me feel more like the person I was always meant to be. But if I barely have time for enjoyable movement, let alone fitness, then my cucumbers aren't going to get the attention they need. Or if I'm not sleeping enough, it's unlikely that I'm going to write in a journal or read before bed.

That's why filling up the bottom levels of the hierarchy matters so much. But once you've taken the time to slowly rebuild your energy, adding core habits and those that enrich, then ideal habits are ready to have a bite taken out of them. Ultimately it becomes a constellation of habits that help support you to be healthy, your best self.

Of course, some ideal habits may feel like they need to come earlier for you. If they're essential for your wellbeing, don't delay! Add them right away. But the reason they're at the apex of the pyramid is because most people tend to start with their ideal habits prematurely, even while they still have gaping holes in their hierarchy. They meal prep, but aren't eating enough to fuel their needs, and are too stressed during to the day to be considered in a well state. Or they keep their scoby alive to brew their own kombucha but miss out on the core food groups. This means they're never really able to stick to the things that light them up and help them feel like their real-est selves. And they're probably not going to be their best self. I don't want that for you. I want you to have ideal habits that are truly sticky.

What is an ideal habit?

In a way, you can think of ideal habits as 'nice-to-have' habits. They aren't exactly essential for being healthy. Think of them like the sprinkles on top of a cake. The problem is that ideal habits are the things that most often get spoken about on social media because they're sexy and fun and inspiring! It can cause you to think they are more important to do than the other stuff. This is how people end up doing *gua sha* but not putting on sunscreen every morning. Or why they take supplements because they're not actually eating a healthy diet. And it's probably what has happened when you buy the latest superfoods, only for them to rot at the back of your fridge (which makes you feel further away from the person you're trying to be).

It's not to say meal prepping or making your own kombucha isn't important; they can be, depending on your lifestyle. It's just that they shouldn't take precedence over more essential habits.

Since becoming a mother, I feel like all I do is pick up shit, so working with manure feels like part of my job description.

Your ideal habits may not be the same as mine. Spending your free time up to your elbows in worms and compost doesn't excite everyone. Each to their own! Your ideal habits are unique to you, and they may (as in, probably will) change during your life, depending on the season you're in.

Ideal habits could include:

* Meditating
* Reading before bed, or anytime.
* Meal prepping ahead of a busy week, even just one dish
* Journalling
* Gardening
* Making food from scratch, such as making bread or yoghurt

How do you work out what your ideal habits are?

Really, it's about getting to know yourself. I know that sounds wishy-washy and a bit intangible but it's doable. A simple place to start is to think about the ideal version of yourself. What things would Ideal You do to look after their wellbeing? Or what do you find yourself doing when you feel like your best, sparkliest self?

Once you've got an idea of your ideal habits, you can quickly run them through the three healthy habits questions to make sure they aren't dieting nonsense in disguise.

Three questions for healthy habits that stick

1. Does this bring me closer to the person I'd like to be?
2. If this doesn't impact my weight, would I still choose do it?
3. Can I do this for the rest of my life?

Then, it's a matter of adding one ideal habit at a time. Trying it on for size. Experimenting. Discarding any that don't seem to fit and building on those that help you feel like the best version of you.

Avoid wellness wankery

There are habits dished out by documentary makers on your favourite streaming service that aren't very helpful. Or Instagrammers who healed their guts by eating air, and now want to sell you an app for $69 a month to show you how to do it yourself. So it's a good idea to ensure that the ideal habits you're creating aren't accidentally wellness wankery.

The nutrition world is filled with misinformation. It's hard to know what to trust. Wellness wankery is fluffy, unscientific advice that does more harm than good. Often, it's based on an inkling of truth. For example, gluten can make some people feel bloated. This small grain of truth is transformed into nonsense, with advice that 'everyone should cut out gluten' or 'gluten is toxic for your gut' (which is all rubbish). Because we notice a bit of a truth to the statements, we find it hard to decipher whether it is something we should believe. You'll have a lot more wellness if you learn to avoid the wankery.

Helping everyone to be healthy without wellness wankery excites me no end. Here are some of the worst pieces of wellness wankery currently circulating on the internet and getting in the way of real health.

Truly, that shit gets me up each day, along with my needy toddler.

The detox myth

Detox teas make you crap yourself and get dehydrated and feel sick. Celebrities who sell you this stuff DO NOT CARE ABOUT YOU. They care about making more money than they know what to do with. The idea of 'toxins' floating around inside us and making us (GASP!) fat are the workings of diet-culture villains. Our bodies detoxify themselves without the help of teas, smoothies or juice cleanses. They actually do a great job of it, because if they didn't, we'd die. The next time you're tempted by the claims of a gorgeous, activewear-clad person who got their qualifications from the University of Instagram, remember this. No juice or powder is going to clear your body of toxins – your liver and kidneys, underappreciated little troopers that they are, along with your skin and lungs will take care of that for you. Save the $300 you'd spend on a detox and do a cooking class or see a health-care professional instead. It's a better investment.

Supplements scandals

Don't spend a stupid amount of money on supplements, serums, potions and elixirs that don't work. There's a good body of evidence behind many supplements, but most people take them when they don't need to, or without expert advice on which is right for them. When this happens, real nutrition experts (food dorks) would agree that it simply becomes expensive pee. And it can place a strain on your liver. And sometimes, it doesn't get excreted and then it's a health problem.

It's just a pH balancing act

Your body does not need help to regulate its pH. It's fully capable of doing that (otherwise, you'd be dead). Please don't waste your money on alkaline water. Simply drink water, and your body will do the rest.

Going gluten free

You don't need to avoid gluten unless you're allergic or intolerant. Most gluten-free food is less healthy, something the wellness world often forgets to mention. Gluten often helps to bind food together, so when it's removed, more sugar or fat may be added to make up for it. If you think you may be sensitive to gluten, make an appointment with a dietitian who can help you healthily manage your symptoms.

Protein powder obsession

Chances are, you don't need to eat more protein. Protein powders are not only an unnecessary expense, they can be problematic because they're often highly processed, and when you eat protein powders you tend to swap out real foods. So why don't you save your money and, let's be real, those nasty protein-shake farts, and eat your protein instead? Oat porridge made with milk contains about 11 grams of protein, one skinless chicken breast 30 grams, three large eggs 18 grams, or a 170 g (6 oz) tub of Greek-style yoghurt about 17 grams. How much protein do we actually need? Women, for example, need 0.75 grams per kilogram of body weight per day: that is, if a woman weighs 70 kg (154 lb), her recommended protein intake is approximately 52 grams.

Ketosis krazy

A keto diet is pretty much just the Atkins diet that has been sold to you again. Intermittent fasting has made skipping meals socially acceptable. Celery juice is expensive pee. Almost all diets work until you realise you can't live on a diet for the rest of your life.

Demonising carbs

Instead of cutting out carbs, cut bad health advice from your diet and you'll be a whole lot healthier. Eat legumes, wholegrains and fruit. Enjoy them, guilt free. Life is better without deprivation.

Essential takeaways

* Ideal habits are nice but not essential, and they definitely come after filling in all the gaps in your hierarchy of healthy habits.
* Many people attempt to add ideal habits without first filling in important gaps lower down in the hierarchy of healthy habits.
* Your ideal habits are unique to you, and they may (as in, probably will) change during your life, depending on the season you're in.
* To make sure a proposed ideal habit is right for you, ask yourself the three questions for making healthy habits that stick.
* Unsubscribe from wellness influencers who spruik misinformation. Check out my podcast for more mythbusting.

Part 3.
Trouble-shoot Common Traps

In Part 2, we talked about how to identify gaps in your hierarchy of healthy habits, and how to collect habits one by one, incorporating them into your life. Part 3 of this book is to help you navigate your way past the traps, mostly caused by diet culture, that make all of this good work way harder than it needs to be. This will help you to be more resilient, less likely to diet and support you to develop real, long-lasting health.

Chapter 13.

Defuse diet triggers

If you want to stop starting a new diet every Monday,
it's important to tackle some of the very real triggers
that can make diets seem like a tempting thing. No, this
time won't be different. So let's build up your strength
to help make you more resilient to diet noise and buffer
yourself from yet another failed attempt.

A number of things can make you want to go on another diet:

* Your mother asking, 'Do you really need to eat that?'
* Jenny from accounting sharing her latest weight-loss triumph or scoffing when she reaches for a 'naughty' snack that will go 'straight to her waist'.
* Someone telling you how awful and guilty they feel after eating exactly same food as you.
* General diet chitter chatter.

Diet talk

If you feel uncomfortable about your weight, have been on countless diets or have a history with disordered eating, it can be really triggering when a colleague or friend or random stranger starts talking about their latest diet. Or bragging about how much weight they've lost. Telling you how bad they feel for eating something. Or nosily enquiring about what you're eating, comparing it with their food.

People who are obsessed with losing weight LOVE to talk about food. And diets. And trade weight-loss tips. If they're on a new health kick, they want everyone to know and comment on how wonderful they are. They assume others are as interested as they are. Plus, they feel it's a socially acceptable thing to talk about.

> Remember that food obsession can be a hallmark of starving people.

At university, I made a really great bunch of friends – the kind of friendship group you think only exists in movies. I was in the peak of my eating disorder (did they know?) and it was agreed unanimously that we were not allowed to talk about diets, food or weight loss in our group (I guess they did know). Or at least they couldn't stand to listen to me constantly bringing every conversation back to food. And perhaps they found it triggering or boring or both. I was deep in the trenches of diet land and can only imagine my constant obsessing about food would have been quite hard for them to deal with.

It was actually a relief for me.

This was the first social group setting where I couldn't fall into talking about weight-loss tips. At my girls-only high school, friends would flock around the lunch table asking me to write up meal plans or dish out dieting advice. I was the go-to person. I guess it was a form of social collateral, my weight-loss obsession and 'tips' I'd gleaned from poring over fitness magazines.

Now, in university, I was talking about other things with my friends. And I think it was a huge, fundamental shift for me. For the first time, I had friends whose connection with me was not determined by weight-loss talk. My brain had to think of other things beyond diets, enough to hold down decent conversations that my friends and I wanted to have together. Slowly, a crack formed in my brain leaving a gap for new thoughts.

If you have a friend who feels the need to weave in diet chat at your catch-ups, you have a few choices: you can continue to see them, though your health feels compromised after each catch up (not recommended); you could stop seeing them as much, casually ghosting them and leaving them feeling confused and unloved (also not recommended); ask them to help you out by no longer talking about diet stuff; or consider suggesting professional support for their relationship with food.

They probably don't realise that when they talk about dieting, it triggers you to feel not good enough, or to want to go on another diet, sending you back swinging on the diet pendulum. And you might be doing them a favour by helping them turn down the dial on diet talk.

Good friends will understand when you say things like, 'Hey, I find it really hard to hear and talk about diet stuff. Do you mind if we make our relationship a diet-free zone? It would help me so much.' You might even have a colleague with whom you can share similar feelings. Put it in your own words. Obviously. And instead of criticism, think of it as recruiting them as allies to help you feel better.

And if they fall into old diet-chat patterns, which they probably will, that's when you swoop in gracefully with a gentle reminder: 'Can we please keep this friendship a non-diet zone?'

Stopping diet talk amongst colleagues is a bit trickier. You can't be as honest. Well, maybe some people can but I'm one of those people with social anxiety who likes to avoid discomfort in group dynamics.

> I am working on this.

Things you can do:
* Talk to the person about it, even if it's just a casual 'food has no moral value' in response.
* Raise it with HR if that's an option.
* Speak to your manager or another team member.

This isn't a guarantee that it will stop. So another thing to do in tandem is to help shift your own thinking about why they are making those comments. Think about it like this. When someone else talks about their weight, your weight, hunger or food, it is a reflection on their relationship with food. It is not a fact. It is not a reflection on your body or appetite. They may be stuck in diet culture. They may not be in a good place and, perhaps, they are where you used to be. Can you have compassion for the place they are at? Personally, I now feel empathy when I hear someone talking like this because I know how much food is still controlling their thoughts.

Trading weight-loss tips and chatting about diets isn't new. In fact, it's something our culture tends to do to connect with others. For my mother and me, it was always something we shared. We would take long drives and if we ran out of topical conversation points we always had food and weight loss to come back to as a point of shared connection and interest. Likewise, there were friends who would happily talk about diets and food for hours with me and it felt genuinely fun! Many of my clients and followers can remember going to group weigh-ins with their mothers or daughters or spending time chatting about diet stuff. It can be something we bond over: a mutual interest, perhaps. But in order to move past judgement around your weight, you will need to sacrifice this topic as a connection point in your relationships.

> An awfully good thing to do; can strongly endorse.

Other diet triggers

When someone else loses weight

This is a hard one. When someone else loses weight, it can be a real trigger to diet. It seems so tempting and doable. Look, someone close to me has done this thing and it's working for them! Before you run out to spend your money on whatever they're eating, first ask yourself, what are they sacrificing in order to lose weight? You can also use the three questions for making healthy habits that stick.

1. Does this bring me closer to the person I'd like to be?
2. If this doesn't impact my weight, would I still choose do it?
3. Can I do this for the rest of my life?

If not, then it's probably just another fad diet.

When others share their guilt

'Argh! I feel like I've turned into a piece of cheese over this holiday!' That's how my friend felt after spending a long weekend enjoying an assortment of yummy cheese plates. I had also spent the weekend eating cheese; was I also a piece of cheese? Should I be feeling guilty for eating something I really enjoyed? Another one is when someone proclaims, 'Wow, I'm so full' after eating just half their plate, while you're still feeling pretty hungry. As we've previously discussed, when people make comments that reveal their guilt around eating, it can feel quite triggering and cause you to spiral into guilt (which isn't very helpful unless you enjoy extreme pendulum swings in your health).

It's very important to be aware that their guilt does not have to become your guilt. You don't have to absorb the pressure they feel to eat a certain way. You may choose to feel empathy for them, knowing they're still working on their relationship with food. Their comments are a reflection of their relationship to food, not something you need to take on board.

Trying on clothes that feel too tight

If you've ever struggled to do up your jeans or felt a roll poke over the top of your pants, you might be familiar with this diet trigger. Feeling uncomfortable in your clothes is a biggie. Let me set this straight: Your weight doesn't have to stay the same your entire life. It's allowed to change. And your clothes should change to fit your body. Your body doesn't need to fit your clothes. I have different clothes for different life stages. If jeans feel too tight, I pop them into a box and store them above my wardrobe until they fit again. If something feels baggy, I keep it because I'll need it again at some point. It gets stored away from my usual clothes. We'll talk about more strategies to prevent body-image stuff from turning into crash dieting in Chapter 15.

Mothers, daughters and food

There is an interesting dynamic that can happen in many mother–daughter relationships. Of course, it's not a phenomenon that's only reserved for mothers and daughters; this dynamic can exist between parents and children of any gender, romantic partners, siblings, grandparents, trusted friends, teachers and more. I refer specifically to it as the mother–daughter dynamic in this book because it is so prevalent in those situations, but please consider how what I'm saying may apply to your relationships, whatever they are.

Mothers can often be the most critical of how our hair, body and clothes look. These constant judgements can be intensely painful. In some ways, we may be wanting to be like our mums, or impress them. So each so-called 'helpful comment' feels like an insult.

The daughter might think: 'This is the one person in the world who is meant to think I am perfect the way I am. But she is constantly finding fault with how I look. I'm never good enough in her eyes.'

From the mother's perspective: 'This is the one person I love the most in the world. I want her to have the best chances at everything and for everyone else to see how wonderful she is. It is my job to support her to be her best self. I only make comments because I love her so much.'

You shouldn't comment on someone else's weight

We're often so willing to sacrifice our health in the name of losing weight. While I was living away from home for university, I once spent a few weeks existing on carrots and barbecue sauce. Strange, bewildering food combinations are a trademark of those with disordered eating. I lost quite a bit of weight. When I returned to my home town, I was praised for how much 'healthier' I now looked. The comments fed me and my eating disorder. By commenting on my weight loss and equating it with wellness, no one was aware that they were endorsing deeply unhealthy habits.

I've spoken to many people who tell me a similar story:

* 'When I see my mum, she can't help but comment on my weight – or tell me all about her latest diet. How can I get her to stop?'
* 'The last time I went to visit my parents, my mom berated me for having a second helping. I was so embarrassed. I ended up crying, leaving early and going to a drive-through on my way home.'
* 'My mum's always made comments about my weight. She thinks she's helping but I hate it. I've asked her to stop but she doesn't.'
* 'My mother-in-law is always on a diet. She loves to talk to me about it, but I hate it.'

Teenagers whose parents comment on their weight are 66 per cent more likely to be overweight or obese as adults.[1] The advice I'm about to share will also work to get them to stop making comments.

They think they are helping by commenting on your weight or body or food. But they are not. Their comments leave you feeling judged, ashamed and nervous to eat normally around them. It can trigger disordered eating habits such as hiding food, binge eating and, sometimes, purging. Perhaps you can relate?

One of my followers said her mum tried to sneak a scale into her apartment. Another told me her mum has been commenting on her weight since she was eight years old. And another follower said her mum tells her that she looked better when she weighed less, even though it required very disordered habits to be that thin.

And I bet most of us can relate to being told to 'pull in your tummy'. While parents often talk to boys about growing strong muscles, they tell their daughters to be careful not to gain weight. That's sad. So let's start to see if we can change that, yeah?

When people comment on your weight or body – or criticise how you look – it can stay with you and affect your self-confidence and relationship with food. It does more harm than good.

The truth is that if someone is commenting on your weight or criticising your body and food choices, it says a lot more about their relationship with food than it does about your size. They may be the one with disordered eating or a troublesome relationship with food. And telling them to stop criticising your weight and stop commenting on your body is one way to make sure they don't continute to pass that on to you.

Your mother's relationship with food

I really feel for women from the baby boomer generation and earlier (and you might belong to his group). They were hit hard by diet culture. Just think: counting calories and points, group weigh-ins, Jane Fonda workouts, weighing out food, Atkins and cabbage soup diets. If they've continued dieting, then there were also the fat-phobic years that followed carb-phobia and now there's sugar fearmongering.

Earlier generations spent their lives being taught that dieting is good. Encouraged. Expected of them. And unlike the younger generations coming through now, they didn't have anyone speaking up against diet culture. Everyone thought it was the thing to do. Then, there wasn't any research, as there is now, showing it leads to weight struggles, poor body image, eating disorders and more. They didn't see photos of women with human, normal bodies in newspaper feeds. In fact, they probably only saw perfectly made-up women in their media.

I believe our mothers, our mother's mothers – and possibly our great-great-grandmothers – have been passing down the same disordered eating and poor body-image lessons from generation to generation. But we will not pass down disordered eating advice to the next generation!

Our mothers' generation is also a generation where a husband may have thought it was OK (it's not) to tell her she looks fat, that her bum is too big, or that she needs to change her outfit before she leaves the house because he doesn't like how she looks.

For me, I find empathy a useful tool to help relieve some anger I feel for past and present comments. Perhaps it can help you too? Maybe your mum was raised thinking her worth as a person depended on her taking up as little space as possible by weighing less. Everything around her – including her friends – has encouraged her to diet and think of food as something to control. If she is commenting on your weight, she is still very much stuck in this harmful world. My heart is sad to think of how food and weight probably still control so much of her thinking.

Firstly, realise that your mum probably went through the same thing with her mum. She might have been told her whole life to stop eating or to pull in her stomach or that she was the wrong size. That is sad to me. Try to imagine your mother being a child or the same age as you and receiving mean, unfair comments about her body. Think about how it might have hurt her and impacted her self-esteem. Without anyone around to help her unlearn what she was taught, she passed it down to you.

I'm not saying her behaviour is OK. But having sympathy for your mum as a child may help you to let go of the resentment. Forgiveness is ultimately about releasing someone else from the burden of your anger. And it can help dissolve some of your anger too.

Plus, your mother is getting older and in a society obsessed with 18-year-old photoshopped models, she clings to the idea that looks are how a woman is valued – and then she puts that on you. No one taught her the essential life lesson that she is more than what she looks like. She grew up in a generation where a woman's looks were her biggest asset.

Luckily, things have moved on. You can help your mum move on too, by learning how to do it yourself – by becoming a role model for her – and becoming someone so self-assured and grounded (and someone who knows that it's not worth sacrificing 95 per cent of your life to weigh five per cent less), your healthy thinking and actions may be passed on.

Your mum may never stop dieting. Or commenting on your weight. Your mum may never change. But you can set clear boundaries and remind her that dieting is an off-limits topic with you. You can lead by example, even if she may not ever 'get it'. You can change how you respond to her comments – and see them for what they are: potential disordered eating and really crummy body image compounded over many years. You can feel grounded in what you now know. Have empathy for her experience. And learn to be more like a duck, letting water roll off its back. What a relief.

You don't deserve to have anyone body shame you – especially not someone close to you, who is supposed to give you care – whether that is your mum or someone else.

Step 1. Set seriously clear boundaries

For you to be able to feel comfortable eating with your family – without fear of judgement – it's important to set clear boundaries about what sort of comments you won't tolerate. You will need to have a conversation with your mum (or whoever makes comments about your weight) letting them know that it is NOT OK. Choose to have this important conversation at a moment that feels best for you.

Here are some conversation points, which you can put in your own words and share with your family.

* When you make comments on my weight or my body, it makes me feel . . .
* I think you say these comments because you're trying to help me but they have the opposite effect.
* If making comments about my body or weight helped, wouldn't I be the weight you want me to be at by now?
* When you comment on my weight or food it makes me feel less motivated. Your comments set me up for an unhealthy relationship with food.
* Please stop making comments like these. It's not OK.
* Do you understand what I am asking you? Do you think you can respect this request? (It's important to get an opt-in agreement so that it's clear what the arrangement is.)
* Hey, I wish I could talk about this but I find it's not great for my mental health.

This conversation might not be easy. There may be tears (or there may be none)! But it's an important one to tackle.

Here are some responses to possible outbursts or criticism:

They say:	You can respond with:
'Do you just expect me to not comment on your eating when you stuff yourself with food?'	'Yes, that is exactly what I'm asking of you. We can't keep trying the same strategy and expect a different outcome. I'm asking you to respect me.'
'You're just going to get fatter if I don't comment.'	'It's my body, so it's my rules. If your comments helped me lose weight, I would have the perfect body by now.'
'People who love you have to tell you the truth because no one else will.'	'If you love me, then you will respect me when I tell you it's not OK to comment on my weight.'
'You asked me to help you lose weight. You wanted me to help you eat less. I'm just doing what you told me!'	'I did ask you to help me because I thought that it would help. But I made a mistake. And now I'm asking you to never comment on my weight or food.'
'It's just a joke! Why are you always so serious? Geez.'	'It's not funny to me. I'd really appreciate you finding something else to laugh about that isn't at my expense.'

Step 2. Reinforce clear boundaries

Here's the most important part of the process. You need to be prepared for the fact that your mum – or another family member – will probably 'forget' that you asked them not to make comments or criticise your weight or body. They may try again.

I can't explain why, but I've learned from experience working with many clients that it takes more than one chat. Perhaps they find it hard to break the old habit. Or they've forgotten about the conversation. Or they're frustrated or are trying their luck. Either way – it's not acceptable.

So when your mother – or another person close to you – comments on your weight again (even after you've told them not to) you need to firmly remind them that it is NOT OK.

Try something like this:

✳ 'I notice that you're [insert offensive thing here; e.g. commenting on weight again]. It's really important to me that you stop these comments. It's not OK.'

✳ 'I asked you not to tell me how much to eat or when I've had enough. My body will tell me how much food I need. I need you to stop commenting on my food and my body. Do you understand what I'm asking you?'

You need to be firm. Especially if you're not a 'firm' type of person – then it'll hold even more conviction.

Sadly, you'll need to keep reinforcing those boundaries as many times as it takes. Argh. It's tedious. I know. Wish you didn't have to. Remain firm. Hopefully, they will finally get it.

Step 3. Don't fall back into old habits of weight talk

After enough time has passed, there may come a moment further down the track when you might want to talk about weight or food with the person again. This might happen if you're going through a period of weight change, or habit change, or learning about yourself. If you do go through this, find other people to talk to about food and your body so that you don't complicate that relationship. If you've gone to the effort of defining the relationship outside the bounds of diet culture, it's best to preserve that safety zone.

Step 4. Lead by example

Whether or not your mother (or whoever it is) stops making comments, there is always the option of leading by example. If you work on creating a role model of a healthy relationship with food, there's a chance that your positive relationship with food will rub off onto them. This will be a great outcome. If you're learning to accept and respect your body – diving into things like intuitive eating – it might become intriguing for them. Be the change you want to see, right?

The food police

Dieters. We have this habit of recruiting people we love and/or respect to play 'food police' or 'weight police', hoping that being accountable to someone will help motivate us. Maybe you once recruited a parent or partner to do this job? Or paid a doctor or nutritionist to do it for you? This strategy can backfire in many ways.

One tricky thing that can happen is it makes you dependent on their presence for discipline. If the only reason you're doing all the things – exercising, eating differently – is to avoid their disapproval, and your subsequent shame, then it's not sustainable. Julie shared her experience with me: 'My doctor weighs me every two weeks, as I need to be accountable to someone who knows what they are doing. Unfortunately she went away for a year and as she wasn't there to watch me I began to put on weight again . . . and then some!' Hmm. Not very sustainable and certainly not something I think is recommendable, even if your doctor is endorsing it.

> Discipline is something, along with willpower, that you don't actually need when you make health enjoyable.

I can relate to this on a personal level. I used to wake at 6 am and drive for one and a half hours to visit a nutritionist for a five-minute appointment, facing a waiting room filled with other people nervously waiting to be weighed and assessed. When it was my turn she would weigh me, then shame me if I had gained weight or react neutrally to weight loss. I paid her very well for the privilege. Knowing I had a weekly appointment meant I was stricter with my diet. But it led to intense guilt and even fear when I deviated from the suggested plan. I was paying someone to scare me into losing weight, a totally unsustainable and disordered thing to do.

Another common trap is recruiting a partner, friend or parent, to 'police' what you eat. This might work temporarily, but it often leads to you finding ways to eat without them seeing. Waiting for them to leave to eat what you really want, crouching in the pantry to avoid the shame of them seeing you, secretly replacing snacks you weren't supposed to have eaten. And then there are the comments you get from them, your food police: 'Should you really be eating that?' or 'Haven't you eaten enough?' But most painful, perhaps, is the sideways look they give you when you veer from your eating plan. Now, not only

Troubleshoot Common Traps

do you feel guilt for 'being bad', but you feel someone else's judgement multiplying the shame. This strategy ends up tying your tricky relationship with food to your relationship with that person, a tangle you want to avoid.

Group dynamics

Perhaps you've entered a weight-loss competition (often camouflaged as a 'get healthy challenge') at your workplace or among friends. Colleagues or mates seem to lose weight easily, while you only become more obsessed with food and then disheartened as you get left behind.

This exact thing happened to Sid, who shared, 'I recently started a weight-loss challenge at my work that required weekly weigh-ins. I think concentrating on my weight each week made me start to obsess again about food. As people around me lost weight at work, I managed to gain around a kilo [2 lb], and started to not like what I saw in the mirror, compared to being relatively happy before. Right now I keep emotional eating and am scared I will keep gaining. I eat a healthy balanced diet and enjoy cooking healthy foods. But because of my emotional eating, I'm finding it hard to feel like I'm in control.'

The opposite can also happen. A group competition drives you to undereat and overexercise, torturing your already strained relationship with food further. A follower called Jenny shared her honest experience with me: 'I started dieting when I looked in the mirror about a year after high school and couldn't figure out when my body had changed so drastically. I remember going on a mission, dumping junk food out of the house and joining a 12-week weight-loss program. I developed a severe case of FOMO with the group of fitness friends I had amassed on social media and if they did a workout I had to workout harder; if they ate something clean, mine had to be cleaner and healthier. I became obsessed with not just how my body looks, but with what I was eating and how many likes it amassed too. Now, almost three years later, I've gained all the weight back, if not more.'

When the desire to lose weight is strong, it's easy to think recruiting a loved one or joining a group will provide motivation. There are a number of reasons why this approach fails us. Apart from the shame or judgement that it can bring, you also end up giving someone else way too much control over your relationship with food.

Plus, instead of being internally motivated (and health motivated) – 'I am doing this because I like how it makes me feel' – you end up with external motivation where the healthy habits can feel like a chore or punishment – 'I have to do this, otherwise I will feel humiliated'. It's an unhealthy, unsustainable and unhappy place to be.

Trauma, shame, food and your weight

Trauma is an emotional response to a painful event.[2] People who have experienced different types of abuse or neglect, or been in terrifying accidents or natural disasters, may carry enduring trauma, sometimes known as post-traumatic stress disorder (PTSD). Scientists and researchers are now coming to realise that the definition of trauma is perhaps a bit wider than we imagined it was. And PTSD can occur in varying degrees of intensity and can be of short or long duration.

If you've experienced trauma, you might notice intrusive, unwanted and distressing memories of the thing that happened and find you have flashbacks of the event, upsetting dreams or nightmares. PTSD may cause an intense emotional or physical reaction inside your body when you are reminded of the event. Avoidance (or numbing) is another key symptom: you might try to avoid thinking or talking about what happened, or avoid people or places or activities that remind you of the experience.

According to one study looking at data for almost 50,000 women (British nurses to be exact), 80 per cent had been exposed to trauma.[3] Of those who had been exposed to trauma, two-thirds reported having one or more lifetime PTSD symptoms.

Research suggests that PTSD symptoms are associated with increased prevalence of food obsession.[4] In fact, being exposed to trauma is a risk factor for developing an eating disorder.[5] Eating disorders are uniquely associated with trauma. There is a link between disordered eating patterns and interpersonal trauma experiences such as emotional abuse or neglect, physical abuse or neglect, and sexual abuse.[6]

If you have experienced trauma, it is a brilliant idea to speak to a mental-health professional by asking your doctor for a referral. If you also notice a turbulent relationship with food, these things may be interrelated and it's useful to bring up. You may also benefit from seeing a specialised eating-disorder dietitian to support you on your journey.

Shame experiences

In some ways, ongoing reactions to shame can be a little like PTSD: strong feelings of shame can be painful and can cause lasting psychological damage. Having shame emotions around your body or eating habits can make it difficult to heal your relationship with food.

A client shared a memory with me; a situation that had been etched into her brain. Even though it had happened 12 years earlier, she said it still replayed in her mind frequently and impacted on her relationship with food now. As a bit of background, she had already spent her life preoccupied with weight and food, and was always trying to 'stay on top of her weight'. It was a lifelong obsession. Here's what happened to her. She was out for dinner with her family while on holiday. She had just finished reading the latest diet book (as she often did) that promised that she would feel satisfied with just three bites of dessert. This felt quite revolutionary for her to be experimenting with, so she was excited to trial how it felt for her.

But while reaching for her second bite, her teenage daughter exclaimed, 'I thought we were meant to be sharing dessert!' In this moment, she felt an intense wave of shame wash over her . . . and since then, it's a memory she can still vividly recall. In fact, that memory of being publicly called out for supposedly eating too much (even though she can rationalise that she wasn't overeating) plays on repeat in her brain. Now, when she eats in public, she is hyper-aware of how much food she is allowed to put onto her plate, constantly worrying that people will judge her for eating too much. The fact that the comment was made by one of her own children made it even more upsetting to her. After all, she'd been taught to believe that mothers are supposed to sacrifice themselves for their children.

You see, small, seemingly insignificant comments made in passing can stick in our minds. Being told we have chicken legs or thunder thighs in primary school. Or an ex who told us our stomach was a problem area. They can influence our relationship with food and ourselves years or decades after the words were first uttered, well after the person who made the comment has forgotten it.

Personally, I have a whole stash of these kinds of memories that replay in my brain on doubtful days. Like the time I was walking along the beach with my family, sticky from the heat of the day and from exercising. I was keen to walk the final length down the beach in my crop top, only to be told by my father that I didn't have the body to wear a crop top on the beach and that I should put my T-shirt back on. My mum interjected and came to my defence but the words were said and have yet to be forgotten.

Or the time I was called Trunchbull after I was awarded female athletics champion for earning first prize in shot-put, discus and javelin. For a young girl desperately trying to be thin and take up as little physical space as possible, this nickname was never forgotten, especially as it stuck around for years.

Miss Trunchbull is the villain and mean headmistress in Roald Dahl's *Matilda*.

Because of what I do, I speak with people almost every day about their relationship with food and their bodies. And very rarely will I meet someone who has managed to go through life without acquiring memories like these. It's more common than not.

If you have shared experiences like this, I want you to know that you aren't alone. In Chapter 15, we'll be talking more about body image. But if you struggle with this I also think speaking to a psychologist is a wonderful thing to do. Try to find someone you connect with; perhaps looking for someone with a special interest in disordered eating or body image is a good way to find them.

Essential takeaways

* A number of things can make you want to go on another diet, from overhearing chitchat about diets, a friend or colleague losing weight, hearing someone else worry about what they've eaten and feeling like your clothes are too tight.
* Becoming aware of the things that trigger you to want to go on a diet is important to help prevent you from getting stuck on another diet.
* We've been passing down a disordered relationship with food and our bodies from generation to generation, historically used as a connection point between mother and daughter.
* Having hard but important conversations to try to change this dynamic can be liberating and very helpful on your relationship with food journey.
* Having people in your life who act as 'food police' can make it really hard to not feel judged about what you eat.
* Those who have experienced trauma are at a greater risk of developing an eating disorder.
* Shame around food experiences and body image can stick with us, contributing to our relationship with food and keeping us stuck dieting.

Chapter 14.

How to exist in the real world and still like yourself

Having a flat stomach won't automatically make your life better, and how you look in a bikini doesn't determine your health status. It's tricky to remember these important details when the world you live in is constantly telling you that you are not enough. But you weren't born hating your body, and you can choose to start to view yourself, and the world, differently.

Diet is traditionally defined as 'the kinds of food that a person, animal, or community habitually eats'.[1] But in the fast-paced world of today, we know it is SO much more than that.

Your diet is made up of:
* what you eat and drink
* who you listen to
* what you watch and read
* who you follow on social media
* what you do professionally and in your spare time
* who you spend your time with

As we know, it's not just about the food you eat, but your relationship to that food that matters a whole bunch. And that's determined by all the thoughts, ideas and beliefs you consume.

Social media

We've already seen the way social media can make you feel exhausted all the time or like you never have downtime. Social media is an energy exchange. It might not feel like it because you're not doing a heap with your body or much thinking, but there's a tonne of processing happening in your beautiful – now very cluttered – brain. When you feel like a rest, the last thing you want to do is look at someone else's highlight reel. For hours each day.

How many hours a day do you spend on social media? Or hours per week? I asked my millennial friends, and was stunned to learn they spend anywhere between three and six hours on their phone each day.

Depending on their profession, many spent most of that time on social media, checking emails or reading the news (usually not good news).

To find out how much time you really spend on social media, open your phone. Go to your settings and look for 'screen time' or 'digital wellbeing'. You'll find a summary of your usage.

This past week, I've spent ten hours on my phone, something I'd like to reduce. And honestly? I'd delete my social media accounts if I could. Really. The irony isn't lost on me that I help people feel good about themselves via my Instagram account @nude_nutritionist on a platform that is fundamentally detrimental for mental health and self-confidence. Plus, the online abuse is decidedly unfun. Everyone has an opinion about how you look or what you do.

Here are some comments I've recently received from internet trolls:

* So why she got a face like a horse with overgrown teeth.
* I wouldn't exactly say she looks the picture of health.
* I have a sudden craving to assassinate all Australian 'experts'.
* I only trust dietitians in bikinis.
* I thought you were meant to be healthy. Why does your skin look like that? Unfollowed.

It's twisted stuff, especially the casual threats of violence towards me and that happen to other women on the internet all the time.

I feel for us, as well as for the next generation. Sadly, they've been forced to turn up on social media in order to fit in, be acceptable, liked. Some particularly brave teens may be able to boycott social media, but there's a lot at stake for those who do. It was hard enough when we were growing up with bullying, teasing and cliques. Now if you make one wrong move, it's on social media for all to see and publicly mock.

It's time to get rid of anyone on your social media feed who makes you feel anything less than amazing and inspired. And be ruthless. Culling those offending accounts is essential. They don't even have to know you've unfollowed them, thanks to the 'mute' function on Instagram. If you want to be kind to yourself, I also highly recommend not using the 'search' function on Instagram (that's the magnifying glass thingy). And you can turn off 'content you may like' from turning up unannounced in your feed.

Unfollowing and unsubscribing from accounts that make you feel bad is a good starting point. But realistically, it's not game changing. The algorithm will always find ways to show you content that you'd prefer not to see. The home feed on Instagram (at the time of writing this) is now a mix of people you follow plus loads of semirelated content from people you don't.

I'll be brazen here. Delete your social media accounts. Or if that feels too wild for now, delete the apps from your phone. I think your life and mental health would likely be better for it. Research backs me up on this one.

We've all done that thing where we decide to use less social media, delete the apps and then approximately 11 minutes later (or a few weeks if you're more stubborn) we're back on. Unlike food, social media is addictive.

There are other ways to connect with people without social media. It's been done before, I've been told by baby boomers.

Some questions to ask yourself:
* Would your mental health be better without social media? Mine would.
* Would you spend less money on things you don't need? Without a doubt.
* How else would you stay connected with others if not through social media?

Last week I bought a specialised ear cleaner thanks to a Facebook ad. I get more packages than text messages.

If the equivalent of blowing up your social media account feels too risky an option for now, what about unfollowing everyone (and every brand) except your real friends. I'm not talking about people you know, but what if it was whittled down to your favourite 20 to 40 people? Would that create more headspace in your life?

A sneaky side note: If I lose all my followers by sharing this advice then I too can finally delete my social media accounts and finally go live in Costa Rica surrounded by sloths and mangoes. See, you'd be doing me and you a favour. Be brave. Delete your social media.

Comparison and jealousy

One of the biggest issues with social media (beyond how it turns you into a compulsive shopper thanks to compelling advertising) is how it flicks on feelings of comparison and jealousy. If you want to remain on social media, but find you get these uncomfortable feelings, here's something to try.

Empathy. Do you really think influencers have it all sorted? I really don't think they are as happy (or self-obsessed) as their curated feeds make their lives out to be. I've met loads of influencers in my time. And, from what I know, influencers – and people who are posting constantly – aren't self-obsessed so much as quite insecure. Seeking validation from a platform that they feel they must turn up on in order to fit into social ideals.

The great actor Alan Alda says, 'I've noticed that the more empathy I have, the less annoying other people are.'[2] Ha! Well, this can also apply to jealousy. Empathy can help you reduce feelings of jealousy (and perhaps how annoying you find certain people) and it's a powerful tool to use.

As soon as I'm able to have empathy for someone (this isn't quite the same as feeling sorry for someone), I notice my jealousy – or annoyance – dissipates. Or at least I can numb it for a while.

Another thing to try is a mantra. I think the idea of a mantra sounds wishy-washy and woowoo, and, while I am yet to accept the word 'mantra', I have started using them and find they really help. My psychologist taught me this one, which I'm practising and enjoying recently: 'I am enough'.

Another one that helped me loads with comparison? 'I accept myself and I accept others.' For me, a mantra acts as a circuit-breaker for the brain, helping me to notice unhelpful thinking and 'change the channel' like flicking the remote control.

When I go into comparison mode, this is my plan:
Step 1. 'This is comparison.'
Step 2. I repeat my mantra.
Step 3. Change the channel.
Rinse and repeat as needed.

The health media you consume

I've been working with the media for ten years now, appearing on TV regularly, doing radio interviews, providing comments and writing articles for print and online publications. It's a strange, imperfect industry. And I think if you understand how health articles are written, it'll help you decipher the BS a little easier.

Recently, a journalist reached out to me about an article for a glossy national health magazine. The story was about how to lose weight, but given that the piece was going to print around Easter, they were worried about the pitchforks that might come out for publishing a food-shamey article near the holiday of the chocolate egg. Could I please contribute some tips to help people ditch guilt related to food (so it can sit side by side with an article about how to restrict)?

You see, since the non-diet movement has gained steam – and now that there is a constellation of those who've realised that hating your body for eternity is cruel and unfair punishment for existing – publications don't want to be seen as promoting disordered eating. They'll publish articles like 'How to be more confident and love your body!' alongside their well-performing weight-loss articles like 'How to lose five kilos in three days' or 'Ways to get a flat stomach'. Is it progress or is it only making things worse?

If you've ever read a listicle promising you '10 ways to lose a dress size in 10 days' or, more commonly, how to curb cravings, take a moment to appreciate that it was likely written by a journalist, not a nutrition professional. And while journalists are typically very lovely and very good at what they do (that is, writing in an engaging way), they aren't health experts. And they aren't immune to the pressure to be thin or have disordered eating either.

A detailed food survey filled out by over 4000 women aged 25 to 45 in the US showed that 75 per cent have disordered eating.[3] That's huge, right? Of the 75 per cent, ten per cent qualified as having an eating disorder such as binge eating, orthorexia or anorexia.

Sadly, disordered eating has become commonplace. In fact, it's so common it has become the social norm. Just

Just because it's common, it doesn't mean it's OK or healthy.

imagine what this means. It means many of the journalists writing our health articles may have disordered eating. Many health-care professionals, nutritionists, health gurus, healers, influencers and even doctors are also likely to experience disordered eating.

The very people we turn to for health advice can be affected by something and not even realise it. I mean, the reason I became a dietitian was because I thought it was the perfect profession to help me stay thin. How messed up is that? It was only through studying nutrition and going through recovery that I realised I wanted to practise differently, helping people break free from disordered eating. You can just imagine how many of the people we turn to for advice are accidentally weaving in their own disordered eating opinions.

I've received emails from tabloid journalists, with a bunch of photos attached of celebrities who are clearly struggling with an eating disorder. The request? Could I please use my university qualifications and expertise to guess the weight of these emaciated, skeletal women? After I pick my jaw up off my work desk and pop my eyes back in their sockets, I write a passionate (read: angry) response where I have to use all my willpower not to include expletives. And you know, that journalist is simply going to find someone who is willing to lower their standards to fulfil the request. The media is powerful and when someone has the chance to get their name in a national publication, they tend to jump at it.

Here's a few more insights into how the health media industry's gluten-free cookie crumbles. A journalist receives a brief from their boss, on a topic they probably don't know all that much about. Their job? Pull together an article within a very tight deadline. Sometimes, a journalist only has a few hours to make magic and get the words on the paper and submitted for review before they're smashing out another article.

With the brief in hand, they'll (hopefully) start googling to find a health expert and the first person who replies to them will probably get the gig. They'll have to trust that health professional to give them the lowdown, and probably won't have a load of time to fact check it (remember, that pesky deadline!). So if someone says they're a 'nutrition expert', they may not have time to investigate their credentials or track record. They'll use their personal judgement but they'll generally take that person's word that they are respectable.

This means that often, a journalist will come to me already with an idea of what they want to write about and the specific angle they're looking for. I might get an email saying, 'Hey Lyndi, I'm writing an article about the best low-calorie Christmas cakes if you're trying to lose weight.' Oh geez. I sigh deeply before pulling up my sleeves and shooting back a counter-pitch, trying to persuade the writer to tweak the angle to be less, well . . . unhealthy, disordered and confusing to the public. I'll try to explain as tactfully as possible. 'That's going to be tricky for me to talk about as calorie counting can make healthy eating harder. Plus, Christmas is a special occasion so I'd recommend people just buy the type they really enjoy, and eat it without guilt. Holidays are about enjoyment, not counting calories!'

But you know what happens then? Unhappy with my response and set on sticking to the brief, they move onto another health expert who is willing to dish out the diet advice they were originally seeking. I might not ever hear from them again. The article still gets published and will be read by hundreds of thousands of people who now think normal Christmas cakes must be avoided for weight loss simply because it exists on a prestigious website.

Generally, I don't think this is really the journalist's fault (though sometimes it totally is). I've worked with plenty of journos before and they're trying to do good, honest work. It's a news and media system that's failing journalists as much as it's failing us. Online, what we click on determines what gets published next. It's supply and demand. Feeding us not on what is factual or good for us but what will get the most eyeballs.

Media used to be quite trustworthy. Newspapers were the source of truth. Journalists had a reasonable amount of time to file their articles. Fact-checking subeditors hadn't been outsourced to AI. But the pace of working in the media has become incredibly quick. As readers, our appetite for news is insatiable. One journalist friend working for a well-known news site was required to write three articles a day, each and every day, to hit her KPIs. I wonder how much fact checking can really be done in that time.

I don't know if you've read a research article before, but they're nuanced! Hard to decipher with weird science lingo. Some types of studies are more reliable than others due to the design, number of participants, biases and conflicts of interest and more. You need to consult someone who knows how to interpret and translate it into human speech. And that's what I aim to do. But even my words can end up getting misinterpreted with click-bait headlines that don't reflect the actual evidence.

For example, I wrote a piece explaining why it's fab to listen to your hunger and practise intuitive eating. I emailed my well-thought-out responses. The heading of the article ended up being 'Why the hunger scale is the key to your dream body'. Argh, no! That isn't what I said. The article was then republished by other sites with headlines like 'How the hunger scale can help sculpt your body'. Other sites kept republishing this content with untrue headlines and I didn't have control over it.

> For clarity, intuitive eating certainly isn't about losing weight and anyone who tries to sell you weight loss and intuitive eating is a diet-pusher.

The crazy thing about all of this? Once it's published on a news site, we assume it's accurate. So the next journalist pressed for time with an irrationally short deadline comes along, grabs the key points from the article (without going back to the source information) and they spit it out again. Like Chinese whispers, the essence of the information gets more jumbled and less accurate each time it's spat out. This is repeated again and again on numerous health sites until we all just assume it must be true! This is how nutrition and health myths are perpetuated, and it's how they reach you.

Here are a few examples of myths given life on the internet:
* Cravings suggest you have a deficiency.
* Breakfast is the most important meal of the day.
* Bone broth will heal your gut.

Can't tell if it's fact or fake? Ask a health-care professional to confirm. And if your spidey senses go off when learning about a weird and wacky health claim, trust your gut. It's probably wankery, not wellness.

Then there's advertising. An online publication – especially one with lots of readers – will sell ad spots on their website and it's a big money maker. Ads are matched to articles with similar topics, using a machine. Machines are smart but not smart enough to realise that being interested in health isn't the same as weight loss. This is how my articles about 'How not to obsess about your weight' are accompanied by scammy, shamey ads promising you can 'Build a bikini body at any age'. There is some human intervention, but it's not working, is it?

Beyond accuracy, shonky media work is contributing to our self-hatred and body-loathing. Bodies (mostly women, but bodies of all genders) are ridiculed. A celebrity can't win. If they gain weight, they're mocked in a tabloid alongside photos of them enjoying their holidays while in a swimsuit on the beach. If they lose weight, they're either applauded or ridiculed for being 'too thin'. The magazine will feign sadness and empathy, claiming to be worried for their health when someone appears to be overcome by an eating disorder. But of course they aren't actually worried for their wellbeing! They know it'll sell copies. The media and the journalists who do this kind of dirty work are the ones driving those celebrities – and all of us – to never feel like our weight is never acceptable.

Taylor Swift famously called out this double standard, at the same time as she admitted to struggling with bulimia. She talked about how impossible the beauty and body standards are. How you're meant to be somehow simultaneously thin all over but still have boobs and a bum. These outrageously unattainable body goals have led to celebrities like the Kardashians getting (and publicly sharing) their multiple plastic surgeries. We now live in a world where plastic surgery is glorified.

The rise of cosmetic surgery

Some startling statistics: in America, there was a 40 per cent increase in plastic surgery in 2021, with 83 per cent of plastic surgeons reporting an increase in bookings.[4] Perhaps the scariest thing is that 79 per cent (up from 16 per cent the previous year) said that people wanted surgery to look better on video conferencing and social media, a trend they labelled 'ZOOM dysmorphia'. In Australia, it's estimated that 90 per cent of cosmetic procedures are performed on people who identify as women, most commonly aged between 35 and 50. Breast augmentation was the main procedure for women, liposuction for men.[5]

I guess this is about the time where I explain that I've had plastic surgery, something I've never spoken publicly about. When I was 19 years old, I had a breast reduction. Yes, my boobs were really big, an heirloom passed down to me from the women of my family. I hit puberty at ten or 11 years old and by 12 years old I was wearing a C-cup bra. But my boobs didn't stop growing for quite a few more years, until I was having a hard time remembering which letter of the alphabet would fit me.

The idea of humongous boobs might not sound all that bad but I was teased at school for it – and hypersexualised. Having big boobs was how people identified me. I was 'the girl with the big boobs' instead of the funny or sporty one or the girl who snorts when she laughs.

And remember, giant-boobed me was also undiagnosed-eating-disorder me. I was still a teenager and this was the early 2000s. The body ideal was set by the Olsen twins, Nicole Richie and Paris Hilton.

By age 19, I'd spent eight years trying to weigh less and make my body fit into the narrow ideals of health. Yes, I was sick of having to wear two sports bras and being teased, sexualised and identified for having big boobs. More than that though, I hated how they made me look. Big. Large. Like Miss Trunchbull. Never petite and small like women are supposedly meant to be.

So I had the surgery. Do I regret it? No, I don't. But I don't know if I would have had the surgery if I didn't have such a bad body image. I sacrificed being able to breastfeed my children, plus there are scars.

Poor body image is fuelling this drastic increase in cosmetic surgery, along with social media and the idea that 'everyone is doing it'. It's becoming normalised. I don't think I'm anti-cosmetic surgery, because my surgery did help me feel better in myself. And people should have full control over their body. But I do think it's driven by the media, and the constant message we receive that we're never thin, pretty or good enough.

Ultimately, we aren't likely to boycott all media and disconnect ourselves from the rest of the world. But knowing the tricks and manipulations behind how media is created can help you smell the bullshit a little easier.

Before trusting everything you read or see, look for these things:

* Experts quoted who have a university degree in the subject matter.
* Links to scientific research.
* No abusive or derogatory comments tolerated by admins.
* A headline that aligns with the article content.
* Less personal opinion, more facts.

Essential takeaways

* Social media is an energy exchange, which may explain why you don't feel rested when you use it as downtime.
* Wellness wankery emerges based on a granule of truth, with misinformation built on top of it, making it hard for us to determine if it's trustworthy or nonsense.
* In the digital age, journalists are being asked to prioritise clicks over facts.
* 75 per cent of women may experience disordered eating. This means that our journalists, doctors, health-care professionals, friends or family may not be immune to diet messaging.
* Not sure if it's wellness or wankery? Ask a health-care professional to confirm.
* Cosmetic surgery is on the rise, at an exceedingly fast pace. Combined with social media filters, what you see on social media isn't a reflection of what people really look like.
* Addressing poor body image and disordered eating before considering cosmetic surgery is a really important thing to do.

Chapter 15.

A guide for bad body image days

A heads-up, dear friend. This isn't going to be some woowoo 'love your body' chapter, throwing another serve of unattainable positivity your way. I reckon we can all buy into the body love stuff up to a point, but we need to tackle the underlying things that stop you from feeling comfortable in your skin. I'm not going to ignore you and those very real, pressing thoughts that get in the way of body acceptance. But here's an alternative way of thinking about it, which I hope you find helpful.

I can't promise that you won't still have some bad body image days. Loving your body in a world that is constantly telling you to weigh less is damn exhausting stuff. It's perfectly normal then (though I wish it wasn't) to have days where you feel like your body is wrong. There will be days when you wake up and don't adore your body or hate how you looked in that photo. The good news is that you don't have to love your body. You really don't. However, your body is worthy of respect regardless of how it looks.

While it's normal to have an occasional bad body image day, when every day or lots of days are bad body image days, that's when you really need to make some changes. For some people, many of the clients I've helped, hating their bodies was a daily occurrence and consumed their thoughts, getting in the way of self-esteem and happiness. This is not the life you deserve. The aim is to reduce the number of bad body image days to a more manageable level (at least in the first instance) so self-doubt is more occasional and, when they do happen, you have the tools to flip the internal dialogue so that it doesn't sabotage your wellbeing.

My hope is that after reading this book, and specifically this chapter, you'll be armed with new skills so that when those inevitable bad body image days happen, you won't fall into the dieting trap.

You'll gain skills to help you:
* practise body acceptance
* bounce back from negative body comments or triggers quicker
* prevent poor body image from derailing your health
* feel less tempted to go on another weight-loss diet ('cause we all know how those end)
* chisel a Greek god out of pure marble with just the nail on your left pinky toe. OK, not this, but everything else can be achieved.

What to do when your confidence is low

I spent many years hating myself (and my body) for being the 'wrong' weight. This has ruined holidays. It's caused me to leave parties early or to not turn up because I felt like I had nothing to wear, while the entire contents of my bursting wardrobe lay on my bedroom floor, with me slumped in the corner trying not to cry.

A number of things would trigger a bad body image day. Seeing my passing reflection in a shop window and looking bigger than I hoped I would. Noticing spiky hairs on my legs and snaggly toenails while I'm meant to be zen at a yoga class. Struggling to pull my pants up over my bum, cursing myself for no longer fitting into my clothes. Catching up with a friend who just lost a tonne of weight and feeling envy that it wasn't me. Or simply eating more than I deemed was acceptable over the weekend, the rising guilt somehow convincing me to undereat to supposedly help balance it all out.

It took me a decade of beating up on my body to realise some very important things. And I want to share them with you.

As we've learned, hating your body doesn't motivate you to get healthy. And it doesn't lead to sustained weight loss. Not in the long term, anyway. When you have a bad body image day, your knee-jerk reaction is to go on a diet or bury your head in a tub of ice cream. You're more likely to resort to unsustainable and extreme approaches to get rid of the feeling as soon as possible. And so, the health pendulum swings wide in response to this unpleasant feeling.

This may lead to trying things like laxative tea spruiked by the internet, even though it makes you shit your pants and feel awful for days. Or buying one of those uncomfortable waist trainers. More wasted money. It means you sign up to yet another 'healthy lifestyle program' that's really just a diet in disguise. And you stay stuck in the same boring cycle of constantly dieting while hating your body.

Hating your body is bad for your health and it doesn't lead to weight loss.

Secondly (and this one is trés important), disliking your body isn't actually a reflection of how worthy your body is. You can quite quickly 'feel fat' moments after finishing a large meal, even though you haven't suddenly gained weight during the 20 minutes it took you to chow through a burger and chips. That's another clue that this feeling is shady and unreliable.

I'm told that many size 0 models report experiencing bad body image days. If hating your body was a true reflection of how it looked, surely those who are thought of as the world's most beautiful people would be free from the self-loathing poor body image brings?

At my skinniest weight, I often had the worst body image. When I see snaps of myself back then, I feel sad for the girl who hated her body. What about you? Have you ever seen an old photo of yourself and thought, 'Wow, I looked so good back then!'? But if you cast your mind back to that time, you can easily remember how you'd wanted to lose weight or change something about your body. Now, with hindsight, you can clearly see that you looked fabulous. How come you couldn't appreciate how amazing you were? Why couldn't you see it before?

That's because a crummy body image isn't based on what you weigh or your body-fat percentage. It's based on your perception of your body. And that perception is manipulated and warped from years of being told that you will never be pretty, liked or thin enough. The problem is that when you hate your body, you believe it. After all, you trust your brain, right? Your brain alerts you when you are cold or need to poop. And it's always right about those things! So when your brain tells you that your body is flawed, you don't question whether society has programmed your thinking to be skew-whiff. You trust that feeling to be 'fact' and accurate.

It's essential to come to terms with the idea that, unlike knowing when it's time to pee, feeling your body is wrong isn't something to attach too much meaning to, especially not your self-esteem or mood. It's certainly not worth jeopardising your mental or physical health.

As I mentioned, only a small minority of people will be able to build up their body confidence to a point where you escape these hating-my-body days completely. For the rest of us, we need to have a plan for noticing bad body image thoughts. The first step is to notice the rising feeling within us. Then challenge the idea that the thought, like 'I am lazy/ugly/wrong', is fact. Facts are permanent and true;

this is really just a feeling, and feelings are temporary and situation dependent. Then, consider what kind act you can do for yourself to help the feeling shift. Personally, I find my mood is almost always improved by moving my body (while listening to my 'body confidence' playlist). Rather than assuming your body is the problem, the thing that needs fixing, consider what else may have caused this feeling. Too tight clothes? That's not your body's fault, but a garment problem. Use the activity on page 268 to help manage poor body image feelings.

A good reason to boycott the expression 'feeling fat' is that it contributes to weight stigma. The implication of the statement is that fat is universally bad, even though you need to have fat on your body to survive. When you say 'I feel fat' to a friend or blurt it out online, it can be perceived as an insult by those who are fat. Or it can lead those with eating disorders to double down on their efforts.

Unconditional confidence

Despite what magazines tell us, real confidence isn't earned by removing your body hair, colouring your brows or finally getting 'toned'. Real confidence can't come off with your waterproof mascara, toupée or Spanx. Real confidence doesn't wilt under a fluorescent light bulb or wither with each birthday cake you receive.

Conditional confidence is a flighty, fair-weather friend. The kind of confidence I dream of for you is much more grand and permanent. That juicy, succulent kind of confidence – the kind that can be felt and seen in someone no matter what they're wearing – is impossible to fake. Real confidence sticks with you. It's unconditional, like the way your parents love you or how you love your children. Unconditional confidence goes everywhere with you, no matter what you wear, where you are in the world or what you weigh.

Many people try to avoid discomfort by trying to build temporary confidence: to cover up insecurities with make-up, get surgery, lose weight or use photo-editing apps. This is a mistake because, to a degree, discomfort is the path to confidence; just as you become more confident at public speaking by getting up in front of an audience and feeling the nerves, breathing through them and learning that even if things don't go to plan, you're still OK.

You won't feel more confident with how you look by covering up all the things you don't like about yourself with make-up or clothes. Well, not for the long term anyway.

Do the things glossy magazines tell you to do and you can temporarily fake confidence, but you won't build unconditional, long-lasting, life-changing confidence – the type of confidence meant for you.

Chasing compliments

Do you do things because you're seeking other people's praise? When we have self-belief and self-esteem, we don't rely on other people complimenting us. When we are doing what we want to, because we're internally motivated, we don't need someone to compliment us.

When we punish ourselves with exercise and restrict what we eat because we're trying to fit in, be more liked, be complimented, we're going into dangerous territory. This kind of motivation – 'I'm doing it for someone else' – doesn't have the stamina. It's short-term motivation that fades once the compliments inevitably peter out. What if we did things because they make us feel good?

I used to be addicted to compliments. I'd put in a lot of effort hoping to be recognised, praised, adored, appreciated. And when the compliments stopped coming, I'd try harder, put in even more effort until I finally got noticed.

I used to wear make-up every day and put a huge amount of effort into my appearance. Because I looked like that all the time, no one complimented me on how I looked, and I really did want those compliments. Without them, I questioned whether I was keeping up with my self-imposed standards. I'd get jealous too, when a friend who usually put in little effort to 'look good' would gain compliments simply because she brushed her hair.

This is a huge difference to the person I am now. No one asks if I'm sick when I don't wear make-up, because that's how I look most of the time (fancy trick, right!)

Are our standards really self-imposed, or was I raised to think my value as a woman was based on how I looked?

The point is, we can't rely on compliments about how we look to give us confidence. That's conditional confidence. It's a flaky confidence that will ghost you faster than that average dude holding up a fish you met on a dating app.

A lot of people seek compliments from others. It's something I hear often in the fitness world. 'Do it for the compliments' was a motivational poster I once pinned to my vision board. There are people whose weight-loss ventures are buoyed by these 'you look amazing' compliments. It's motivating. And I know that first hand.

But if you want to get healthy and stay there, you really need to NOT do this for the compliments. It must be for yourself. Because once you reach your goal, those compliments will dry up. You'll be putting in all this effort and no one will notice and those compliments that once propelled you forward and played a role in why you did the healthy things won't be there any more.

Embrace unconditional confidence

You aren't born with confidence and you can't buy it. While some people have natural talent or good looks, confidence is something you build and cultivate with time and practice. And once you've developed real confidence by doing it through practice, it's comforting to know that it can never be taken away from you.

To get unconditionally confident, you need to:
* learn to be cool with being imperfect
* allow yourself to be average and awkward and odd
* realise you're always a work in progress

You probably weren't born hating your body. Watching my toddler play, I'm in awe of how unfiltered he is. He isn't at all self-conscious and judgemental. When we play in the bath together, he isn't judging my body or his own. He is simply existing, enjoying learning – free from thoughts about not being good enough. This is because he's too young to understand the pressures we all have from society.

Your body is imperfect, and it always will be. Can you choose to accept that about yourself and free up your headspace for other things that will make you happier? I think accepting your body is a choice, a decision you make in spite of what your body really looks like. This isn't about giving up on how you look or not having pride in your appearance. It's about simply accepting that no matter how hard you try, you will always be a work in progress.

Can you forgive your body?

A question for you: can you forgive your body when you do all the 'healthy things' and it still doesn't look the way you hoped? If you want to live a full life, you're probably going to have to accept that your body will never look perfect. What I'm saying is, yes, be healthy. Do the things that make you healthy – get sleep, eat vegetables, cook at home more, drink water – but when you do these things and your body STILL doesn't look the way you wished it would, it's time to forgive it.

You don't have to love your body

I don't believe 'loving your body' is the goal (though it's great if you get there). Making the leap from body-loathing to self-love can be too grand a movement to make in one go. The aim is to get to a point where the flatness of your stomach doesn't dictate your self-worth.

* **Body neutrality:** not really focusing on your body or how it looks at all, acknowledging that it's not a determinant.
* **Body acceptance:** accepting that your body is imperfect but still choosing to care for it.
* **Body respect:** regardless of how it looks, choosing to give your body respect.
* **Body love:** loving your body regardless of how it looks or any perceived imperfections.

I want to be strong and feel comfortable in my body. But I don't think I could get rid of cellulite on my tush and a protective layer of fat on my stomach without sacrificing my life or getting bogged down in food obsession. This is what I need to accept in order to live a full life.

Being pretty or thin is not the best thing you can do

No one is going to talk about how thin or pretty you were at your funeral. No one will say, 'They changed my life because they were so skinny.' While that helps put it in perspective, I get the battle. Everything around us makes us feel like being pretty and/or thin is an impressive thing. But if you think of all the time and energy you spend on the pursuit of liking yourself through manipulating how you look, you could spend that precious headspace and time on much grander pursuits. You could do a whole number of things that would flabbergast others and, most importantly, yourself.

No one really fits in, anyway

One of the reasons we do all of this diet stuff is to fit in, right? To be liked. Accepted. Appreciated. To finally feel worthy enough. To some degree, we can all relate to the feeling that we don't quite fit in. Even the cool kids, the people you think have it all, they feel this way, too. You may even be that person who others think has it all and yet you can't shake the feeling that, mmm, you don't really have your 'people'.

The magic of self-compassion

You're already good enough. You deserve to be treated with love and respect. You know that deep in your bones, right? But there's also a mean girl (or person) in your head, talking shit about you, things you would never say to anyone else. Imagine your brain as a radio: when you hear that negative voice, change the channel from self-loathing to self-acceptance, because the latter is way more enjoyable to tune into.

Let's work with some examples here. I start by simply telling myself:

* 'It's not my life's purpose to have a flat stomach and look good from every angle.'
* 'I'm exactly where I'm meant to be.'
* 'I accept myself – and I accept others.'
* 'My body is allowed to change. I trust that my body will look after me if I listen to it, instead of criticism.'

If you had to choose between your ideal life or your ideal body, what would you choose?

I won't spend the rest of my life hating my body

Gerry heard this statement and practised doing it for themself. They shared with me, 'I cannot keep counting and tracking and punishing myself with exercise that I hate. This more free way of eating and just moving my body in ways that I enjoy is so much better for my mental health. Although I am still working on the mindset of losing weight, I am reminding myself that I am putting lots of nutritious food into my body and moving every day and that health is the ultimate goal.'

Yes! Because your body is allowed to change during your life. It's incredible if we think back to how much we've sacrificed to chase a body we never seem to be able to reach and maintain.

Do healthy things, move in a way that is enjoyable . . . it's freeing to know your body doesn't have to be perfect in order to be healthy.

* I don't need to eat perfectly in order to be healthy.
* Healthy enough really is good enough.
* I am imperfect. And so is everyone else.

Aim to be a horse, not a unicorn

We are expected to be fit and funny and fashionable and organised and sexy and spontaneous, but can we really be all these things? There will be things that you are good at, but there will always be someone smarter, prettier, more put together than you. Striving to be special is exhausting. It's alienating. Disconnecting you from others.

If the goal is to be happier, to have better relationships, to be healthier, then let's accept that we are horses. We can do hard work and be admired. Be strong and capable. You don't need to try to be a unicorn, a mythical, unattainable creature.

This doesn't mean you have to settle, or stop trying. It means you can give yourself a break, forgive yourself for not being able to reach the mythical goals you've been set. It's lonely at the top, striving to be something that doesn't even exist. It's OK to be a horse, not a unicorn.

Why you have nothing to wear

In the height of the pandemic lockdowns, it felt like every day I was receiving a new delivery of clothing. While wide awake at 2 am (thanks to anxiety and a newborn), I'd be scrolling through fashion sites. In a way, I was trying to buy happiness, to make myself feel better in a world that felt miserable and overwhelming.

Constantly buying new clothes is more than just wanting to have stuff. It's a symptom of hating your life or your body. It's rooted in poor body image and not liking the version of yourself you see in the mirror or in awkward photos taken by a friend. The thought? Buying new clothes is going to help me like myself more. But it's a temporary high. Compulsive shopping is a self-esteem issue, more than anything. It can be a symptom of crummy body image. And rooted in the thought that other people are better, prettier, happier than us.

After giving birth to my baby, my feet grew by a whole size. As annoying and expensive as it was, I didn't hesitate in buying new shoes. I didn't blame myself or my body. I didn't force my feet into the smaller pairs that no longer felt comfortable. I didn't think it was my body's fault that my feet were broader and longer than before. Being unattached to size is easy when it comes to shoes: we buy the size that fits. But we don't do the same thing when it comes to clothes.

Many wondrous, seriously smart people I meet are buying the wrong size clothes, convinced that it'll motivate them to lose weight. I've certainly done this. Purchased a dress that I thought would look better if I weighed less, kept it and then never felt comfortable enough to wear it. Or kept items I hoped to fit back into one day.

The impact of this is a closet bursting with clothes while you're left with the feeling of 'I have nothing to wear' or 'nothing looks good on me'. I've seen fashion stylists attempt to solve this problem by suggesting a capsule wardrobe or defining our style (all good things, I would agree) but, when it comes down to it, this nothing-to-wear phenomenon is often a body-image and self-esteem issue more than anything else.

Beyond the mental fatigue that comes from never feeling quite comfortable in your clothes, there's the impact it can have on your eating. If you wake up and getting dressed feels like it triggers you into self-loathing, one of two things could happen. You either decide to go on an extreme unsustainable diet (and we all know how that ends) or you end up emotionally eating to help you feel better. Don't underestimate the power of having clothes that fit you.

This is the story of my client Maureen. 'I found a photo of myself when I was 18 and skinny as a rake, but I had a little pot belly. Guess it's my body shape! I suddenly realised on Sunday that the weight and body shape I'm at now is obviously what I'm meant to be. It seems that every time I lose weight, six months later I'm back here at this weight! It has only just dawned on me that this is my body's sweet spot and I'm learning to be happy with that. I am still working on the mental side of things as well as learning to normalise food, but I think after years of yo-yo dieting, I didn't know what I was supposed to look like. I'm healthy and reasonably fit and that's something to celebrate, not feel disappointed because I don't fit into my "skinny" clothes anymore. It's amazing how good it feels to wear clothes that fit properly and aren't too tight.'

Newsflash: clothes need to change to fit your body. Your body doesn't need to change to fit clothes. What if getting dressed could be enjoyable, or at the very least, not trigger you into a day of hating your body and then the subsequent diet-thinking that follows?

If you find it's impossible to get dressed in the morning – if it triggers you to hate your body, which drives you to emotionally eat – your wardrobe, not your body, is what needs to change. It's time to buy new clothes, in a different size. You deserve to feel comfortable in your body. Here are some strategies to try on for size.

Do not buy clothes that you need to lose weight to feel comfortable in

I can't tell you how many times I've done this and it's a waste of money and depressing. You might think, 'If I had the right underwear, this would look a lot better' or 'If I lost a bit of weight, this would fit really nicely'. Buy clothes that fit you now. It's important. You deserve to wear clothes that you feel good in now. The alternative is that you end up with a wardrobe that doesn't fit or make you feel as brilliant as you deserve to feel.

Check the time

Recently, my husband and I went to a flashy, fancy dinner spot to celebrate ten years of being together. I squeezed into a sexy, black body-hugging dress I felt fabulous in. While waiting under a fluorescent light for our ride to pick us up, a homeless man congratulated me on my pregnancy.

'No, sir, I'm not pregnant. I've just eaten a 14-course dinner' was my response (or at least it was in my head).

You see, I probably could have sized up on this dress, something I only realised later on. But because I'd gone shopping for this LBD in the morning, I hadn't taken into consideration how I'd feel wearing it in the evening, following a big luscious meal.

As the day goes on, as we eat, move and breathe and live, it's natural and normal for your stomach to distend a bit. So be smarter than I was when I made this purchase. Before buying, consider this: when did you last eat? What time of day is it now and what time of day will you likely wear this outfit? Therefore, if you're buying a form-fitting dinner-party dress first thing in the morning, to ensure you're comfortable in that garment, you'll want to check there's enough room for digestion and general tummy expansion.

Are you a T-shirt fluffer?

There's a shared habit amongst people who feel body conscious: T-shirt fluffing. It's when you're sitting down and feel the need to fluff or reposition your top so that it's hiding your stomach – or any other part of your body you feel uncomfortable about. Or you subsconsciously place a pillow or your bag over your stomach to hide it.

We all do a bit of T-shirt fluffing – it's only normal – but frequent fluffing may be a sign that your pants or skirt are too small, making you feel self-conscious about the normal phenomenon of stomach rolls. Or your top doesn't make you feel comfy as it should. Notice if you have to regularly tug at your clothes to feel more confident.

Order online

For some perplexing reason, the lighting in retail stores is deeply unflattering. I can't explain it! So if you can, get clothes delivered to your house so you can try on items in the comfort of your home where you have access to the right underwear and normal lighting. These days, it's become quite a seamless process to shop online.

Try being unposed

We all do this thing when trying on clothes we're thinking about buying. We pose, trying to look our best to determine if this garment deserves a place in our wardrobe. The problem with this is that it's the equivalent of taking a selfie on your camera (a cute photo where you can pick the angles that make you feel good) versus the photo someone shares on social media where they look great but you look like a pudding.

Of course, do the posing thing in front of the mirror for the try-on but then take a moment for some non-posed moments. Are you pulling in your stomach? Are you flexing or twisting in a certain way? Try standing normally and comfortably – you might even go for a short walk – as this is likely how you will look out in the wild while wearing these clothes.

Do the sit-down test

According to my mum, some shoes are 'sitting shoes'. These types of shoes are misguided purchases that are perfectly fine to wear while seated but transform into torture devices while walking. Not ideal when you consider the purpose of a shoe! The same applies for clothes. Almost always when trying on clothing, you are standing. Stationary. Striking a pose.

It's a really good idea to change this up. In the fitting room or after you've dressed, make sure you sit down. Can you comfortably sit in these clothes or are they too tight and uncomfortable? Notice any desire to fluff your clothes to 'fix them'. And notice any 'If I . . .' statements like, 'If I had the right bra/lost some weight/pulled in my stomach/wore smoothing underwear/didn't have my period I could wear this confidently.'

Could you wear this item on a day when you're feeling less confident or is it an item that requires you to be in the right mood? After a meal? The same thing applies to trying on bras as your relaxed chest is a different formation from a standing, posed chest. Do the sit-down test to see if the garment deserves a place in your closet.

✎ Breaking the bad body image cycle

Hating your body isn't good for your health. The obvious reason is that it mucks with your mental health, but bad body image can also lead you to waste money, time and energy on quick-fix diet attempts, exposing yourself to those rubbish consequences. You can have the best intentions, but if you have a nagging voice in your head saying 'you need to lose weight', it's going to be hard to let go of diet rules or adopt truly health-focused habits. Here's a step-by-step plan for dealing with bad body image feelings.

Step 1. Notice when you're experiencing poor body image.

You might notice a desire to lose weight, or feeling sad about your body. When you start to feel your thoughts drift into self-loathing, can you start by noticing the negative self-talk pattern.

Step 2. Acknowledge what triggered the feeling.

When you notice that you're in the throes of shaky body confidence, the niggling 'my body is awful' thinking starts clouding your brain and your thoughts turn to ideas of dieting, it's really useful to become aware of what triggered you to feel that way. Try to identify what made you feel bad about your body; it could be any number of things.

* Someone making a comment about your weight, or failing to comment on your weight if you were hoping they'd notice a change.
* Seeing a photo of yourself where you don't like how you look.
* Catching a glimpse of yourself in the reflection that you don't consider to be flattering.
* Putting on clothes that feel too tight.
* Seeing a friend, colleague or acquaintance who has recently lost weight.
* Not getting enough likes on a photo you posted on social media.
* Looking at photos of beautiful people, while scrolling the internet or flicking through a mag.

This is a common pattern for how feeling triggered can lead to assumptions about weight, leading to dieting behaviours.

Trigger: Seeing a photo of yourself when you look bad.

Thought/feeling: Bad body image/hating how you look/feeling fat.

Emotions: Feeling sad, disappointed and angry with yourself.

Behaviour: Planning to diet, promising to be good.

Step 3. Translate what that really means.

Fat isn't a feeling. What you're feeling is discomfort in your body based on all the things you've been taught to think about your body. Ask yourself: What would help me feel better right now?

* Realigning with my hierarchy of healthy habits.
* Going through my wardrobe, throwing out clothes that don't fit.
* Spending less time on social media.
* Going for a walk or exercising.
* Putting on clothes that make me feel good about myself.
* Reminding myself I don't need look perfect to be happy or healthy.

There are a number of things you can do to feel better in your body. With time, you'll learn which strategies work the best for you. You can keep these in your back pocket so that when poor body image moments strike, you'll be less likely to be derailed and can push back against the insecurity.

Essential takeaways

* You don't need to love your body. But can you choose to show it respect, or view it neutrally, accepting it will always be imperfect?
* You don't have to look perfect from every angle. In some photos you'll look fabulous, while other times you'll look like a pudding. This isn't a reflection of your self-worth, because being pretty or thin is the least impressive thing you can do.
* Managing bad body image days starts with recognising the thought patterns. Poor body image is a feeling, not a factual assessment. Consider what triggered the feeling, and do something proactive that can help you move through it.
* Grow unconditional confidence, not flaky confidence that depends on compliments from others or your weight.
* Can you forgive your body for not being perfect?
* Change your clothes to fit your body, don't change your body to fit your clothes. Your wardrobe can either support you to feel good in your body or get in the way of your wellbeing. Changing your relationship with clothes may help shift your relationship with your body.

Chapter 16.

Raising healthy kids who like their bodies

In the social media age, our children are more vulnerable than ever to damaging health messages and body image pressures. Even more than we were when we were littlies. Eating disorder rates are on the rise, for boys and girls, and non-gender conforming children too. It's scary.

While you sadly can't prevent them from absorbing the constellation of things that tell them that there is something wrong with their natural body, you can prepare them with a tool belt of strategies to help buffer the impact. And hopefully protect them by building their food knowledge and teaching them body respect and coping strategies.

This chapter shares serviceable pointers for parents and guardians, grandparents, aunties and uncles, and those who care for little ones. So we can help our kids grow up to be healthy with better self-esteem than perhaps we were given as children. Raising children to have a healthy relationship with food can set them up for a lifetime of healthy habits, sparing them the torment of thinking their bodies are intrinsically flawed. It's big stuff. It's important stuff. Let's dig in.

Dieting starts way too young

What age did you start dieting? My client Kelly started too young. She explains, 'I have had a bad relationship with food since I was about five: the age I was put on my first diet. It didn't work. I remember getting in trouble late one night because my mum found me eating apples I'd stashed during the day in the bathroom. I have been body shamed by my immediate family, extended family, old work colleagues and strangers.'

Girls' beliefs about dieting and weight are often learned from their mothers. In a study conducted in 2000, young girls aged five years old whose mothers had recently dieted were 50 per cent more likely to have ideas about dieting. And of the mums who were interviewed, 90 per cent of them had recently dieted.[1]

The grim news is that research has shown children may begin to worry about weight and appearance as young as ages three to five,[2] and that many kids express unhappiness about their bodies. But while as a parent you can choose how you approach weight and body image with your children, it can feel like a touchy subject with family.

Like for adults, diets don't work at reducing body weight for young people. Not only don't they work, but they can lead to a bunch of crappy mental-health outcomes like eating disorders, depression and feelings of worthlessness.

In research from 2015, 60.5 per cent of UK teens exercised specifically to lose weight, a big increase from 6.8 per cent in 1986.[3] Over a ten year period, a great proportion of adolescents were trying to lose weight: 42.2 per cent, up from 29.8 per cent in 2005.[4]

More young girls thought their weight was 'about right' when they were categorised as underweight according to their BMI (60.8 per cent in 2015, compared with 42.3 per cent in 1986).[5] The same study found that teens who diet for weight loss are significantly more likely to have depressive symptoms.

While young girls have always tended to be more preoccupied and aware of weight pressure, children of all genders are now feeling the pressure to engage in weight-loss behaviours.[6]

It's concerning stuff. Especially when 44 per cent of 14 year olds reported dieting in 2015.[7] That's a huge number, especially when you consider the harm. Not only do diets not work but they are associated with weight gain, depressive symptoms, feelings of worthlessness, self harm and eating disorders.[8]

And kids who end up dieting? Well. They can get set up for a tricky, turbulent and unhealthy relationship with food as they get older.

There are currently one million Australians living with an eating disorder, according to The Butterfly Foundation.[9] My own disordered relationship with food and my body started at age 11 when a nutritionist put me on a calorie-restricted diet because I was bigger than other kids.

Josie told me, 'My first recollection of dieting or being concerned with my weight is from when I was about eight or nine. I can remember trying to hold my stomach in to look thinner; feeling self-conscious at my tenth birthday about my top/skirt combination. My first real "diet" was in Year 8 or 9: I would "challenge" myself to not eat on a Friday at school, and I was proud when I got to 4 pm and had intense hunger pangs. Another was when I spent about three months on a strict "fruit salad and frozen yoghurt for morning tea and salad roll for lunch" diet, and straying was not an option.'

A study from 2017 called '"Don't eat so much": How parent comments relate to female weight satisfaction' revealed important insights that can help us raise our children to respect their bodies.[10] Of more than 500 women who participated in the research, those whose parents made comments about their weight reported that were more likely to struggle with poor body image. And they were also more likely to have a higher BMI. And regardless of BMI, women were more likely to feel dissatisfied with their body if they remembered their parents commenting on their weight.

A wonderful follower called Trish shared her story with me: 'My mum put me on my first diet when I was 12, but I remember my weight being talked about before that point. My entire adult life has been a cycle of disordered eating. It wasn't until I had my own children that I realised how damaging it had been.'

It is possible to comment on your child's food intake without impacting their body image or having a negative impact on their weight as an adult.

The most powerful tool you have as a parent is to set an example

Ooofff. I know. This is a biggie. And it's not easily done or won. It might be the very reason you're reading this book. Perhaps like me, you grew up believing that your body needed fixing and this cascaded into a lifetime of body-loathing and chronic dieting. Like my client Imma who said, 'I've been yo-yo dieting since my teens, tried beyond absolutely everything. I'm almost 40 and still struggle with weight and food but desperately want to be a good role model for my two-year-old daughter.'

If you're motivated to work on your relationship with food and your body for your children's sake (as much as your own sake), I applaud you. With a standing ovation. Call me biased but, as a dietitian, nutritionist and mother, I reckon teaching kids how to eat – something they will do multiple times a day for the rest of their life, something that will impact their quality of life, mental health, immunity and self-esteem – is a seriously important thing.

Unlike sponges, they tend to make way more mess than they clean up.

Children are sponge-like in how they absorb and learn everything that they can from you. One thing you can do starting today is updating your food language. This will have flow-on effects for you and them!

Update your food language

Using healthy food language around children is so crucial for them developing a healthy relationship with food. Research from the *Journal of Nutrition Education and Behavior* shows that mothers of heavier children use different words to restrict eating than parents of children with smaller bodies. Parents of children with obesity were more than 90 per cent more likely to use direct statements such as, 'You're only allowed one more' to prevent children from eating high-energy 'sometimes' food as opposed to other mothers who used less direct statements like, 'You have had dinner'.[11]

Small changes can quickly help you update the language you use around food. It's nuanced! And tricky. One thing you can do is stop referring to food as 'good' or 'bad'. That's because the words 'good' and 'bad' are intrinsically loaded with moral value, and applying those judgements can be unhelpful. And if you can, try not to use food as treats or even call them 'treat food', as this can create an emotional relationship between their mood and what they are allowed to eat.

Sometimes, when talking to our children, we can say things absentmindedly that we don't quite realise could be triggering or unhealthy for their relationship with food or their body.

Phrases you might say to your kids without realising

* 'Did you really just eat all that food?'
* 'How can you still be hungry?'
* 'Do you really need to have dessert?'
* 'Wow, you're really eating a lot today!'

Instead of saying these phrases, you could use these moments as opportunities to help them be better guided by your appetite.

You could say:

* ✶ 'How does your tummy feel? Are you still hungry?'
* ✶ 'If you're still hungry, then that's your body's way of telling you to have more.'
* ✶ 'Do you think you're hungry or is it just really yummy?'

If your child is older and saying these things would feel too strange, see if you can notice your child's appetite but don't feel the need to comment on it. Be a role model by eating when you're hungry. It's important not to make them worry that there is something wrong with their appetite simply because you think they're eating more than you think they should. Remember, you've got years of dieting under your belt, so trust that their appetite is a reliable guide for them. Even if they do overeat, allowing kids to do so is part of them understanding their appetites.

Allowing kids to experience that sick-from-eating-too-much feeling builds your child's internal feedback loop so they can learn for themselves that 'when I eat too much chocolate, I don't feel good'. This is critical. We want our kids to be able to listen to what their tummy says, because as adults, we've often lost track of our internal hunger management system – our appetite.

Given some independence around food, children will likely self-regulate. As parents, if we can get out of their way, help them listen and respond to their body's innate cues, they will develop an internal motivation to eat well. When they become adults, this can transform their thinking from, 'I shouldn't eat too much chocolate because it's bad for me' to a much healthier perspective of, 'I don't want to eat too much chocolate because it doesn't feel good'.

So the good news is you can save your energy, worrying each time they reach for another snack. Yes, it might be tempting to jump in with phrases like, 'Eat your greens, then you can have some chocolate' or 'You've had enough', but try not to interfere.

We want our kids to learn that chocolate is just food, and they can eat it without becoming obsessed with it. After all, research suggests parents who place too much control over discretionary foods like chocolate can contribute to children having a long-term obsession with these foods.

There's room for all foods in a balanced diet

Kids who have regular access to all foods can choose to eat as much as they feel like and stop when they've had enough – that's intuitive eating. It's unhelpful to categorise foods as 'good' and 'bad'. While there may be foods that are healthier than chocolate, this does not make chocolate a 'bad' food that deserves feelings of shame or judgement when enjoyed.

As for bribery, as a mother of a toddler I'm not above it, but food-as-reward can be a slippery slope to emotional and binge eating. I'm not keen on planting the idea that some foods have to be earned, as I know first hand how this can lead to the opposite idea – that eating those foods must be followed by 'working them off' or, essentially, 'earning' them after the fact. Instead, I prefer to offer non-food based rewards like some time at the park or an extra book at bedtime.

Talk about how food makes you feel. Not weight.

When we're worried about our child's weight, it's tempting to encourage them to eat less. But even well-intentioned comments can have long-term negative consequences for our kids. A woman's dissatisfaction with her adult weight is related to the extent her parents made comments about her weight.[12] It's something I know from my own experience. Research shows that 66 per cent of teenagers whose parents comment on their weight will go on to be overweight or obese.

One study showed grown women whose parents had commented on their weight were far more likely to have a higher BMI and dislike their body.[13] In fact, the more comments they received, the more weight they gained. Research also suggests weight-based comments make you far more likely to develop an eating disorder.[14] Other studies show that weight comments encourage binge eating, emotional eating and eating in secret or hiding food.[15]

When talking about food, never talk about eating certain food because it will make you fat or help you lose weight. Instead, talk about how food makes you feel and what it does for you. Explain that some foods give us great energy so we can do the things we love like play with friends and do sports. You can explain that some foods make us feel better than others. Teach them to eat all the colours of the rainbow to get all the nutrients to grow strong and healthy.

Zoning in on what our bodies can do rather than what they look like is a really nice lesson for kids. Whether it's how strong their arms are, how fast their legs can run, how deep their lungs can breathe, how clever their brain is, all these things can help build a positive body image that has nothing to do with thinness or size.

Teaching kids about appetite

Remember being taught to finish everything on your plate? This advice teaches children to ignore natural hunger and appetite cues. Teach your children to tune into their hunger. Explain that hunger is a way of telling us when we are ready to eat and fullness is our body's smart way of telling us it's time to stop eating. If they aren't hungry, don't force them. If they want food, ask them if they are hungry or bored or tired or something else? If they are hungry, let them fill up on as much healthy, everyday foods until they feel full, while not restricting them from less healthy options either

It might mean one day they graze on next to nothing and the next eat for the world, but our appetite is the key to feeling normal around food. Your appetite's purpose is to provide energy for your body, which is unique and different from others.

I quite like the phrase, 'Oh, you're having a hungry day' when I'm speaking to my son, said in a neutral tone. It feels like I'm helping him to understand that some days he will naturally be more hungry, and other days, less hungry. The tone really matters, and so does the age of your child. The opposite, 'It seems you're just not as hungry today', comes along with it so that there is balance showing the natural ebb and flow of appetite during growth spurts, teething, busy daycare or school days and whatever else.

However, I can see how saying, 'Oh, you're having a hungry day' to a tween or teenager is going to hit them quite differently! Sounds confusing? That's a fair assessment. As children become more aware that thin is the idealised body state, accusations that they are eating too much or too hungry (no matter how you phrase it) may teach them that there is something wrong with their appetite.

Just one more bite!

Dinner time with kids. You used at least three different vegies (hello colour!), dressed them up with some delicious cheesy sauce and are about to start your own home-cooking channel, you're so pleased with yourself. That's until your kids turn their nose up at what you've served. What is this rainbow dinner when all they want is a beige buffet? Frustration sets in. You believed this was one meal your kids would enjoy. Why did you waste your time – and food? But while it's tempting to start a dinner-table power struggle, threatening that they must eat it or at least have one more bite, it's not a good idea.

'Please. Just have one more bite . . .' is a plea uttered by many desperate parents at meal time.

As a parent of a toddler, I understand it's easy to feel worried when your child isn't eating well or concerned they'll go to bed hungry. So what harm is asking them to have just 'one more bite' when it's encouraging more variety in their diet?

As parents, we just want what's best for our kids – and with 95 per cent of Australian children not getting the recommended amount of vegetables a day, it's easy to fear they're not filling up on the healthy stuff.[16] The big problem with the 'one bite' rule is that it's a rule, and associating rules with food is never healthy. It moralises food and can lead to guilt and shame. Encouraging a child to eat more or less than their appetite says they need can disrupt their internal feelings of hunger and fullness. It's a big problem we see today with so many of us eating by the clock, or a meal plan, rather than by appetite.

Bottom line is that the eating habits you start as a kid go with you into adulthood. Creating pressure around food can lead to children ignoring their natural cues. Of course, we need to remember kids have very little control in their lives. Where they go, what they wear, what they are going to eat is largely determined by us, so they often flex their independence in terms of what options they choose to eat.

Strategies to encourage picky eaters

Ask yourself, would I actually eat this? When it comes to kids we can sometimes go too purist or 'clean' with food. Plain can also mean devoid of flavour and fun. If what you're serving your child seems unappetising even to you, then it's time to rejig your thinking and try out some different recipes. Shameless plug: finding new, kid-friendly recipes doesn't have to be tricky. My app Back to Basics is designed for busy parents and people who just want a yummy, easy and healthy dinner sorted.

Play dress-ups. This isn't about adding sugars and salts, but adding flavour to food. Olive oil and cheese are two versatile options, while I like to add peanut butter to broccoli so it's not so sad and doubles as an allergen exposure.

Try up to ten times. We want our kids to eat variety, so while it's easy to feel despondent, don't give up. Research shows children often need at least ten times of seeing a new food before they'll even try it, whereas we as parents tend to give up after three to five exposures. Given the effort and waste – it's understandable – but persevere if you can. Simply place the food on your child's plate (a small amount to start). Even if they don't touch it, this small interaction with the food counts as an exposure.

Combine with familiar foods. Introduce a novel food along with a food they already accept. If pasta is much loved but zucchini isn't in favour just yet, use a peeler to create zucchini ribbons. Or add zucchini to some pasta sauce. Or try grating just a touch on top.

Role model. Sit with your child and eat bits of the same food you served to them. It's not about tricking them, but showing you enjoy carrots too. And if you don't? Find another healthy option you do enjoy.

Batch cook and freeze. Use ice-cube trays to make small portion sizes so you can continue exposing new foods to your kids without huge waste. This also gives you the option to keep changing things up and present new food without making it the whole meal. By giving small amounts, kids still have their familiar favourites, while not getting overwhelmed by the unknown.

The way you speak to your child now will inform how they will eventually speak to themselves. You're helping to shape their own inner critic, to hopefully be, well, a lot less critical. A gift every kid deserves to unwrap. An inner voice that speaks kindly and gently.

Raising imperfectionists

How you talk about other people matters. Judging and commenting on other people's bodies, appearance or food intake can be harmful. If you judge other people, what they eat, how much, their weight or things like how attractive or intelligent they are, your kids will notice.

Firstly, it teaches children how to judge and compare themselves to other people. Suggesting that beauty is a contest, that there is always more that could and should be done to improve. The sunset is beautiful and so is the willow tree. One isn't more beautiful than the other. They are just different.

Secondly, it teaches children that people are very judgemental. I mean, the world is very judgemental so I guess this is a fair thing to know. However (and it's a BIG however), raising kids in a judgemental immediate environment amplifies this fear. The fear that 'everyone is always judging me'. A child thinks, 'I don't want to be judged' so they aim to do everything perfectly in an attempt to avoid the discomfort of judgement. They strive to become perfectionists. Because when you grow up in a judgemental environment, you come to believe that being perfect is what is expected of you, even though it's a completely unattainable goal for anyone. And so you get set up for a lifetime of striving for something that you can never have. For perfectionists, there is no destination.

Can we help prevent our children from becoming perfectionists? Yes and no. Certain personality types and specific traits can lead someone to perfectionist thinking. But there is an environmental factor, a role that the family unit can play in helping to reduce the pressure. Try to notice and stop yourself from judging other people. You might still have the thoughts. I mean, humans are pretty intrinsically judgey. But can you practise noticing those thoughts without verbalising them, especially while children are in earshot?

Here are some examples of scenarios to be aware of.

✱ Notice the comments you make about the people you see on TV and their appearance. Try not to comment on the news anchors' hair and make-up, or whether they've gained weight or lost weight.

* When you run into an old friend or acquaintance. If they look different from how you remembered, can you avoid making a comment about them while you drive away from the encounter with your children in the car?

Resist the urge to judge yourself. And others.

Your children listen closely to everything you say and do. This means that if you're complaining about your body, they'll pick up on it. Making comments about how much you hate your body, certain body parts or complaining about your stomach rolls or that you overate will teach children that this is how you should talk to yourself.

I know it's not easy to feel comfortable in your skin. But it's worth working toward.

Step one? Simply become aware of your own self-talk. Step two? Try to practise speaking kindly to yourself, especially in front of your children. You'll teach them to see what's incredible in themselves. Your children will see you enjoying a dessert, along with everyone else, exercising for enjoyment and eating bright and colourful vegetables at meals.

What to do when others make body comments around your kids

Even the most well-intentioned comments can have long-term negative consequences on our kids. Have people made 'innocent' comments like these to your kids?

* 'Look at your cute fat little tummy.'
* 'You shouldn't eat that. It's fattening.'
* 'You've hit the puppy-fat stage.'
* 'You wouldn't want to get fat, now would you?'
* 'Don't you think you've had enough?'
* 'You've got such nice skinny legs.'

If you're a parent, and there's someone in your children's lives who is likely to make negative body or food comments in front of your kids, it could be a chance to recruit them as an ally: although it's not always possible and sometimes tricky. Especially if it's a mother-in-law who often declares, 'I'm so fat!' in front of your little ones even after you've had several chats. In Chapter 13, we've already covered ways to ask people kindly to stop making these sorts of remarks. It's worth doing the same for your kids, as children tend to role model after the people they spend time around.

Here are some things you can do:

1. Pre-empt things. If you were raised in a weight-centred, body-shamey, dieting household (I'm sorry; that sucks) your kids will likely encounter comments about weight from your family. Instead of waiting until something is said and making an example of it, consider a proactive conversation. It could cover how you're raising your kids and what language you'd be appreciative of your family using. Chances are they don't even realise what they're saying can be harmful.

2. Recruit them. There's nothing to be gained by a 'he said', 'she said', so by asking for mindfulness you can recruit them to be allies, rather than critique what they have done. It's nice to be on the same team. Get them onside early. Find your own words, but you could try something like, 'We'd love to raise our kids with a positive body image. Can you please support us by not commenting on their weight, bodies or food intake? And can you also please not comment on your weight or other people's bodies around them? That would be so appreciated.'

You can explain that kids who receive comments about their weight are 66 per cent more likely to be overweight or obese. Plus it sets them up for a complicated, unintuitive, all-or-nothing approach to food. Be firm and stay firm. It's important for your child's health.

3. Offer gentle reminders. And realistic ones. This won't be a one-and-done conversation. From my experience, I've needed to reiterate the message many times before change has happened. Be kind. Remember it's easy to slip into old habits, so be prepared to gently remind them as many times as needed.

You can't control everything. There are going to be times when bad body talk shows up in your child's life, whether it's through the

Troubleshoot Common Traps

conversations they hear, books they read or TV shows they watch (even shows designed for children can sometimes be a bit body shamey, so I'd suggest watching episodes together, or choosing more inclusive shows).

How you feed your children is a reflection of your relationship with food

Since becoming a mother, I noticed something interesting. How I feed my son, well, it's a reflection of my own relationship with food. Do I treat him with food when I feel he's done something tough?

I admit I find myself doing this. If we're out and I want him to stay calm so I can have a moment of adult chat, I'll give him something to nibble on. He isn't really hungry: he didn't ask for food. But sometimes, it's easier to throw food at our kids when we need a well-deserved moment.

> If you have a pet, you might notice the same thing happens.

Common advice is not to bribe kids with food, or use it as a reward for compliance. But what about this other stuff? Feeding them to prevent them from being bored? To buy us time as adults? Or to use it as a soothing method.

Here's what I know. Being a parent is a shit-fight. We're all just trying to get through the days, some of which are terribly long and hard and tear-filled (my tears and theirs!). Suggesting you never do these things, I think, feels a bit unattainable for most of us. If you don't, godspeed and go forth! But for the rest of us mere mortal parents just stumbling through the day, what shall we do?

First up, you can notice when it's happening. For example, I might think to myself, 'He's not actually super hungry right now, but I'd like a moment to sit in this café without him turning into a pterodactyl.' Acknowledging our behaviours and patterns without judgement is pretty much always the first step for most things.

> Unless it's spray tanning, in which case, the first step is always exfoliate!

Simply noticing when you're doing these things might help you rejig your thinking a wee bit, so perhaps you will do it slightly less often. Or you can plan to meet up with friends at a café or during your children's normal meal time so that they can eat while they are hungry. That way they are not eating because they're bored, with fewer occasions for food to be offered simply as an edible distraction toy.

And, if not, then we can listen to them as they naturally adjust their eating afterwards. If my son isn't hungry for his next meal, instead of making him sit down to eat and telling him to 'eat your vegetables' or 'just one more bite', I'll simply ask him if he is hungry. If he isn't, that's all right. I'm OK if he doesn't feel like eating at this moment because he isn't hungry. Yes, even if it means he doesn't have dinner, if his body has enough energy for the day, all is fine. Tomorrow he might eat more. The body helps to regulate these things for appetite.

Of course, context matters. If this is happening every day and your child is eating a croissant instead of a nutritious dinner, then it's time for some tweaking. And if a doctor or paediatric dietitian has advised you otherwise, stick to their advice.

Tips for raising healthy kids who like themselves

Eat at the table, not in front of the TV.

This is a hard one, I know. But this habit starts as a kid and stays with you. Children who eat at the table, instead of in front of the TV or a device, are a lot more mindful of their food and are less likely to keep eating once they are full. Can't commit to this fully? Keep eating in front of the TV for special occasions, like when mummy really needs to lie down.

Model healthy living.

Whether you've got a toddler or a teenager, creating healthy food habits starts at home. Sit down for regular family meals where you can; serve a variety of healthy foods and snacks; be a role model through your own relationship with food; avoid battles or loaded language around food; and involve kids where you can – whether that's grocery shopping or cooking.

Create a healthy environment.

When kids have access to healthy options at home, and see their parents eating healthily, it's easier to stay healthy. Fill the house with fresh, healthy options and that's what your children will eat. If they open the pantry and see chocolate or lollies, it will trigger their brain to crave those foods, even if they weren't thinking about them before. But that said, healthy doesn't mean devoid of chocolate or chips. There is balance. Helping them to understand a healthy balance by what food is available is helpful.

Troubleshoot Common Traps

Get kids involved as much as possible.

Often children get stuck doing crappy, boring chores like setting the table (which is fine) but doesn't instil a sense of excitement about food time. If you can, get your kids involved in the fun side of meal times, like meal prep and shopping. Let them choose fruit for their lunchbox. Let them pick a vegetable they've never tried from the produce section and cook it together. Ask them to mix in the salad dressing on a salad or add the ingredients to the bowl.

Essential takeaways

* Role modelling healthy eating and a positive relationship with food and your body is the most powerful thing you can do to support your children to be healthy and like themselves.
* Avoid the temptation to make shaming comments about your weight, the appearance of others and their bodies.
* Support kids to tune into their own internal hunger and fullness cues, helping them eat when and as much as they need to thrive. Don't force kids to have another bite and try not to let meal times become a battleground.
* Recruit allies to help protect children from body and weight comments.
* Creating a healthy environment for children to grow up, one that supports them to make healthy choices without you needing to control what they eat, can be good for your relationship and their relationship with food.
* Get kids involved in fun, food-related activities rather than making them set the table. Try asking them to pick a recipe, choose a new fruit to try from the grocery store or help you flavour a meal.

Well, it's the end of the book...

But I hope it's the start of your new, healthier relationship with food. Before I leave you, here are some big-sister tips you can store safely under your pillow.

When you live in world that's constantly telling you must weigh less in order to be worthy and happy, it's natural to be tempted to return to the siren calls of old diet ways. The most important thing is to let go of weight-loss goals and focus on your health instead. As long as you hold onto the faulty thinking that 'trying to lose weight leads to sustained weight loss', you'll most likely stay stuck.

Know this. Your weight is not the problem. It's really not. The real problem is how you've been taught to fixate on your weight. And how that's led to obsessing over calories, pounds and how your body looks rather than how your body feels. It's led to an unhealthy relationship with food. Trying to 'fix' your weight by focusing on weight loss is like putting a bandage on your pinky toe to cure a headache. Quite frankly, it's pretty dumb. Hasn't worked before, won't work in the future. Let's remedy the real problem by changing the way you think about eating, weight and your body.

Instead of weighing yourself, eating for weight management or trying portion control, what if you listen to your hunger, work on reducing emotional eating and adopt healthy habits bit by bit . . . until one day you look around and find you're living your healthiest life. The irony is that you may naturally lose weight as a result of doing all these things.

While I hope you've experienced many delightful 'a-ha' realisations while reading this book, it's outrageously important to remember this. If you've been dieting for years – maybe even decades – it's going to take more than reading a book once over (even a very excellent one like this) to transform your relationship with food. Intuitive eating can be a bit tricky to get started with as you learn to trust your body again. But unlike diets which get harder and harder to

Tune into my podcast *No Wellness Wankery* if you want extra support with this new approach.

stick to, this approach gets easier and easier with time! And you
what? You will stumble! You're allowed to 'mess up'. Veering off co
is all part of the process. Be gentle with yourself when you do. Beca
imperfect action really is better than no action.

Realistically, it's a whole heap easier to do this whole no-diet and
love-yourself thing when you've got the right professional support.
To help you get closer to your happily-ever-after relationship with
food, I've got hundreds of free blog posts, recipes, short courses and
book resources available for you on my website *lyndicohen.com*. And
because I've also personally been there, done that, I really care deeply
about helping you reach food freedom.

At the core of it, this approach is really just a process of about
getting to know yourself: learning which foods and types of movement
make your body sing; understanding your unique hunger cues and
patterns; and trusting what works for you so you can confidentiality
ditch the rest. Rather than subscribing to a one-size-fits-all meal plan
(that actually fits no one), think of it as unlocking your own unique
health road map.

So, it's a mighty good idea to keep a record of what you learn.
When you make a few changes that feel excellent for you, please make
a note of it. Squirrel it away in a notepad to serve as a reminder later.
We often think we'll remember these habit shifts, but having written it
down can be really helpful to look back on during moments of doubt.
When the familiar urge to just 'go on another diet' pops up, you'll have
your own personalised road map helping you return to real health.
And you so deserve that.

Big love,

Lyndi
XXX

It takes a village

I'll never accept an Oscar so this is my grand shot at an acceptance speech – and I'm going to milk it! First up, big thanks to the glorious team at Murdoch Books for elevating health experts above wellness influencers: you're my kind of people. A extremely special thank you to my publisher Julie Mazur Tribe for very kindly guiding me to write the best book I could, even when the path to getting there was curly. To my dependable editorial manager Justin Wolfers who always trusted my vision, thank you for letting me run with my big, crazy ideas, even at the last minute. Melody Lord, you've been such a brilliant teacher and trusted editor yet again. Thank you for polishing my words to make me appear more put together! Sarah Hatton, I so appreciate how you've bolstered me and helped me get this book's message as far and wide as possible. And of course, big thanks to Jane Morrow – and Lou Johnson – for always believing in me and the world I'm desperate to help create.

When I started my business ten years ago, it was just me posting painfully average, grainy photos of my breakfast to Instagram and sharing blog posts with plenty of typos. Things have been seriously upgraded since then, thanks to my very clever team. Martina Dietrich, life and work is better because you're in it: I'm one of your biggest fans. To my *No Wellness Wankery* podcast co-host Jenna D'Apice, thanks for 'getting it', you smart, warm human. You're both much loved.

And to the brilliant word-wizards who've helped me craft my message so it's not just ranty (well, at least not all the time), a huge wallop of gratitude goes out to you. Melissa Shedden, you impress me in everything you do. Some people can't help but dazzle and you're just that. Bek Day, you're someone I'd like to be more like. I just think you're brilliant, and quite frankly, I'm in awe of your beautiful brain. To my divine photographer Luca Prodigo, thank you for always making me feel so comfortable, whether you're shooting me six weeks after giving birth, in a bikini, make-up free or cellu-lit. You're a real find.

Lastly, I've got a very impressive bunch of humans supporting me through triumphs and meltdowns as well as uneventful fold-the-washing moments too. To my husband Les . . . as my wonderful late Bobba said to me, 'You couldn't do better if you tried.' And she's was so right. You're all the good bits and you make everything better. Thanks for being the best supporter and partner. To my tremendously loveable son Leo, being your mum helps put everything in perspective. And to the little girl growing in my belly, I can't wait to raise you to truly like yourself. And lastly, thank you to my entire family. To my mum Elize Polivnick for raising me with such love. Now that I'm a mother, I really appreciate everything you've done for me. Hopefully I keep becoming more and more like you. Finally, a special mention to my much-loved late father Dennis Polivnick, I wish you were still here and could have read this book. I know you'd be so very proud.

References

Introduction

1   Hall KD, Kahan S. Maintenance of Lost Weight and Long-Term Management of Obesity. *Medical Clinics of North America*. 2018 Jan;102(1):183–97. doi.org/10.1016/j.mcna.2017.08.012

2   Patton GC, Selzer R, et al. Onset of adolescent eating disorders: population based cohort study over 3 years. *BMJ*. 1999 Mar;318:765–68. doi.org/10.1136/bmj.318.7186.765

3   Hall. Maintenance of Lost Weight and Long-Term Management of Obesity.

PART 1
Chapter 1

1   Booth HP, Prevost TA, et al. Effectiveness of behavioural weight loss interventions delivered in a primary care setting: a systematic review and meta-analysis. *Family Practice*. 2014 Dec;31(6):643–53. doi.org/10.1093/fampra/cmu064

2   Fildes A, Charlton J, et al. Probability of an Obese Person Attaining Normal Body Weight: Cohort Study Using Electronic Health Records. *American Journal of Public Health*. 2015 Sep;105(9):e54–9. doi.org/10.2105/AJPH.2015.302773

3   Hall. Maintenance of Lost Weight and Long-Term Management of Obesity.

4   University of North Carolina at Chapel Hill. Three Out Of Four American Women Have Disordered Eating, Survey Suggests. *ScienceDaily*. 2008 Apr. sciencedaily.com/releases/2008/04/080422202514.htm

5   Siahpush M, Tibbits M, et al. Dieting Increases the Likelihood of Subsequent Obesity and BMI Gain: Results from a Prospective Study of an Australian National Sample. *International Journal of Behavioral Medicine*. 2015 Oct;22(5):662–71. doi.org/10.1007/s12529-015-9463-5

6   Rosenbaum M, Leibel RL. Adaptive thermogenesis in humans. *International Journal of Obesity*. 2010 Oct;34(0 1):S47–55. doi.org/10.1038/ijo.2010.184

7   Grodstein F, Levine R, et al. Three-Year Follow-up of Participants in a Commercial Weight Loss Program: Can You Keep It Off?. *Archives of Internal Medicine*. 1996 Jun;156(12):1302–6. doi.org/10.1001/archinte.1996.00440110068009

8   Foster GD, Wadden TA, et al. Psychological effects of weight loss and regain: a prospective evaluation. *Journal of Consulting and Clinical Psychology*. 1996 Aug;64(4):752–7. doi.org/10.1037/0022-006X.64.4.752

9   Ulen CG, Huizinga MM, et al. Weight Regain Prevention. *Clinical Diabetes*. 2008 Jul;26(3):100–13. doi.org/10.2337/diaclin.26.3.100

10   Mann T, Tomiyama AJ, et al. Medicare's search for effective obesity treatments: Diets are not the answer. *American Psychologist*. 2007 Apr;62(3):220–33. doi.org/10.1037/0003-066X.62.3.220

11   Neumark-Sztainer D, Wall M, et al. Obesity, Disordered Eating, and Eating Disorders in a Longitudinal Study of Adolescents: How Do Dieters Fare 5 Years

Later?. *Journal of the American Dietetic Association.* 2006 Apr;106(4):559–68. doi.org/10.1016/j.jada.2006.01.003

12 Ikeda JP, Lyons P, et al. Self-reported dieting experiences of women with body mass indexes of 30 or more. *Journal of the American Dietetic Association.* 2004 Jun;104(6):972–4. doi.org/10.1016/j.jada.2004.03.026

13 Field AE, Austin SB, et al. Relation Between Dieting and Weight Change Among Preadolescents and Adolescents. *Pediatrics.* 2003 Oct;112(4):900–6. doi.org/10.1542/peds.112.4.900

14 Siahpush. Dieting Increases the Likelihood of Subsequent Obesity and BMI Gain.

15 Neumark-Sztainer. Obesity, Disordered Eating, and Eating Disorders in a Longitudinal Study of Adolescents.

16 Lowe MR, Doshi SD, et al. Dieting and restrained eating as prospective predictors of weight gain. *Frontiers in Psychology.* 2013 Sep;4(577). doi.org/10.3389/fpsyg.2013.00577

17 Thomas SL, Hyde J, et al. 'They all work...when you stick to them': A qualitative investigation of dieting, weight loss, and physical exercise, in obese individuals. *Nutrition Journal.* 2008 Nov;7(34). doi.org/10.1186/1475-2891-7-34

18 Pelchat ML, Schaefer S. Dietary monotony and food cravings in young and elderly adults. *Physiology & Behavior.* 2000 Jan;68(3):353–9. doi.org/10.1016/s0031-9384(99)00190-0

19 Anguah KO, Syed-Abdul MM, et al. Changes in Food Cravings and Eating Behavior after a Dietary Carbohydrate Restriction Intervention Trial. *Nutrients.* 2019 Dec;12(1):52. doi.org/10.3390/nu12010052

20 Wegner DM, Schneider DJ, et al. Paradoxical effects of thought suppression. *Journal of Personality and Social Psychology.* 1987;53(1):5–13. doi.org/10.1037/0022-3514.53.1.5

21 Marketdata LLC. The U.S. Weight Loss Market: 2022 Status Report & Forecast. *Research and Markets.* 2022 Mar. researchandmarkets.com/reports/5556414/the-u-s-weight-loss-market-2022-status-report

22 Finkelstein EA, Kruger E. Meta- and Cost-Effectiveness Analysis of Commercial Weight Loss Strategies. *Obesity.* 2014 Sep;22(9):1942–51. doi.org/10.1002/oby.20824

23 Keys A, Brožek J, et al. *The Biology of Human Starvation* (2 vols). Minneapolis: University of Minnesota Press, 1950. psycnet.apa.org/record/1951-02195-000

24 Epstein LH, Carr KA, et al. Long-term habituation to food in obese and nonobese women. American Journal of Clinical Nutrition. 2011 Aug;94(2):371–6. doi.org/10.3945/ajcn.110.009035

25 Thomas. 'They all work...when you stick to them'.

26 Hall. Maintenance of Lost Weight and Long-Term Management of Obesity.

27 van den Berg P, Neumark-Sztainer D, et al. Is Dieting Advice From Magazines Helpful or Harmful? Five-Year Associations With Weight-Control Behaviors and Psychological Outcomes in Adolescents. *Pediatrics.* 2007 Jan;119(1):e30–7. doi.org/10.1542/peds.2006-0978

28 Istituto Neurologico Mediterraneo Neuromed IRCCS. Pasta is not fattening – quite the opposite, Italian study finds. *ScienceDaily.* 2016 Jul. sciencedaily.com/releases/2016/07/160704101101.htm

Chapter 2

1   Kuijer RG, Boyce JA. Chocolate cake. Guilt or celebration? Associations with healthy eating attitudes, perceived behavioural control, intentions and weight-loss. *Appetite*. 2014 Mar;74:48–54. doi.org/10.1016/j.appet.2013.11.013

Chapter 3

1   Eknoyan G. Adolphe Quetelet (1796–1874)—the average man and indices of obesity. *Nephrology Dialysis Transplantation*. 2008 Jan;23(1):47–51. doi.org/10.1093/ndt/gfm517

2   Nuttall FQ. Body Mass Index. *Nutrition Today*. 2015 May/June;50(3):117–28. doi.org/10.1097/NT.0000000000000092

3   Gruzdeva O, Borodkina D, et al. Localization of fat depots and cardiovascular risk. *Lipids in Health and Disease*. 2018 Sep;17(218). doi.org/10.1186/s12944-018-0856-8

4   Donini LM, Pinto A, et al. Obesity or BMI Paradox? Beneath the Tip of the Iceberg. *Frontiers in Nutrition*. 2020 May;7(53). doi.org/10.3389/fnut.2020.00053

5   Trestini I, Carbognin L, et al. The obesity paradox in cancer: clinical insights and perspectives. *Eat and Weight Disorders – Studies on Anorexia, Bulimia and Obesity*. 2018 Apr;23(2):185–93. doi.org/10.1007/s40519-018-0489-y & Lennon H, Sperrin M, et al. The Obesity Paradox in Cancer: a Review. *Current Oncology Reports*. 2016 Jul;18(56):1–8. doi.org/10.1007/s11912-016-0539-4

6   Donini. Obesity or BMI Paradox? Beneath the Tip of the Iceberg.

7   Gaesser GA, Angadi SS. Obesity treatment: Weight loss versus increasing fitness and physical activity for reducing health risks. *iScience*. 2021 Sep;24(10):102995. doi.org/10.1016/j.isci.2021.102995 & Thomas. 'They all work...when you stick to them'.

8   Pojednic R, D'Arpino E, et al. The Benefits of Physical Activity for People with Obesity, Independent of Weight Loss: A Systematic Review. *International Journal of Environmental Research and Public Health*. 2022 Apr;19(9):4981. doi.org/10.3390/ijerph19094981

9   Strohacker K, Carpenter KC, et al. Consequences of Weight Cycling: An Increase in Disease Risk? *International Journal of Exercise Science*. 2009;2(3):191–201. pubmed.ncbi.nlm.nih.gov/25429313

10 Zhang Y, Hou F, et al. The association between weight fluctuation and all-cause mortality. *Medicine*. 2019 Oct;98(42). doi.org/10.1097/MD.0000000000017513

11 Quinn DM, Puhl RM, et al. Trying again (and again): Weight cycling and depressive symptoms in U.S. adults. *PLoS ONE*. 2020 Sep;15(9). doi.org/10.1371/journal.pone.0239004

12 Ouerghi N, Feki M, et al. Ghrelin Response to Acute and Chronic Exercise: Insights and Implications from a Systematic Review of the Literature. *Sports Medicine*. 2021 Nov;51(11):2389–410. doi.org/10.1007/s40279-021-01518-6

13 Thomas. 'They all work...when you stick to them'.

PART 2

Chapter 4

1   Watson NF, Badr MS, et al. Joint Consensus Statement of the American Academy of Sleep Medicine and Sleep Research Society on the Recommended Amount of Sleep for a Healthy Adult: Methodology and Discussion. *Sleep.* 2015 Aug;38(8):1161–83. doi.org/10.5665/sleep.4886

2   Reynolds AC, Appleton SL, et al. Chronic Insomnia Disorder in Australia. *Sleep Health Foundation.* 2019 Jul. sleephealthfoundation.org.au/news/special-reports/chronic-insomnia-disorder-in-australia.html

3   Pross N, Demazières A, et al. Influence of progressive fluid restriction on mood and physiological markers of dehydration in women. *British Journal of Nutrition.* 2013 Jan;109(2):313–21. doi.org/10.1017/S0007114512001080

4   O'Connor DB, Thayer JF, et al. Stress and Health: A Review of Psychobiological Processes. *Annual Review of Psychology.* 2021 Jan;72(2021):663–88. doi.org/10.1146/annurev-psych-062520-122331

5   Warburton DER, Bredin SSD. Health benefits of physical activity: a systematic review of current systematic reviews. *Current Opinion in Cardiology.* 2017 Sep;32(5):541–56. doi.org/10.1097/HCO.0000000000000437

6   Deng F, Li Y, et al. The gut microbiome of healthy long-living people. *Aging (Albany NY).* 2019 Jan;11(2):289–90. doi.org/10.18632/aging.101771

7   Curtis GL, Chughtai M, et al. Impact of Physical Activity in Cardiovascular and Musculoskeletal Health: Can Motion Be Medicine? *Journal of Clinical Medicine Research.* 2017 May;9(5):375–81. doi.org/10.14740/jocmr3001w

8   Sharma A, Madaan V, et al. Exercise for Mental Health. *The Primary Care Companion for CNS Disorders.* 2006 Apr;8(2):106–7. psychiatrist.com/read-pdf/24919

Chapter 5

1   Dombrowski SU, Avenell A, et al. Behavioural Interventions for Obese Adults with Additional Risk Factors for Morbidity: Systematic Review of Effects on Behaviour, Weight and Disease Risk Factors. *Obesity Facts.* 2010 Dec;3(6):377–96. doi.org/10.1159/000323076

2   Gardner B, Lally P, et al. Making health habitual: the psychology of 'habit-formation' and general practice. *British Journal of General Practice.* 2012 Dec;62(605):664–6. doi.org/10.3399/bjgp12X659466

3   Cameron J. *The Artist's Way* (25th anniversary edition). New York: TarcherPerigee, 2016

4   Leonard JA, Lee Y, et al. Infants make more attempts to achieve a goal when they see adults persist. *Science.* 2017 Sep;357(6357):1290–4. doi.org/10.1126/science.aan2317

5   Conrad DF, Keebler JE, et al. 1000 Genomes Project. Variation in genome-wide mutation rates within and between human families. *Nature Genetics.* 2011 Jun;43(7):712-4. doi.org/10.1038/ng.862

Chapter 6

1   Chaput JP, Dutil C, et al. Sleep timing, sleep consistency, and health in adults: a systematic review. *Applied Physiology, Nutrition, and Metabolism.* 2020 Oct;45(10):S232–47. doi.org/10.1139/apnm-2020-0032

2   Ibid.

3   Ibid.

4   Ibid.

Chapter 7

1 Hill AJ. The psychology of food craving*: Symposium on 'Molecular mechanisms and psychology of food intake'. *Proceedings of the Nutrition Society.* 2007 Apr;66(2):277–85. doi.org/10.1017/S0029665107005502

2 Holt SH, Miller JC, et al. A satiety index of common foods. *European Journal of Clinical Nutrition.* 1995 Sep;49(9):675–90. pubmed.ncbi.nlm.nih.gov/7498104

3 Hill AJ, Weaver CFL, et al. Food craving, dietary restraint and mood. *Appetite.* 1991 Dec;17(3):187–97. doi.org/10.1016/0195-6663(91)90021-j

4 Hill. The psychology of food craving*.

5 Weingarten HP, Elston D. Food cravings in a college population. *Appetite.* 1991 Dec;17(3):167–75. doi.org/10.1016/0195-6663(91)90019-o

6 Ibid.

7 Parker S, Kamel N, et al. Food craving patterns in Egypt: comparisons with North America and Spain. Appetite. 2003 Feb;40(2):193–5. doi.org/10.1016/s0195-6663(02)00160-5

Chapter 8

1 Crum AJ, Corbin WR, et al. Mind over milkshakes: mindsets, not just nutrients, determine ghrelin response. *Health Psychology.* 2011 Jul;30(4):424-9; discussion 430-1. doi:10.1037/a0023467

2 Spiegel K, Tasali E, et al. Brief Communication: Sleep Curtailment in Healthy Young Men Is Associated with Decreased Leptin Levels, Elevated Ghrelin Levels, and Increased Hunger and Appetite. *Annals of Internal Medicine.* 2004 Dec;141(11):846–50. doi.org/10.7326/0003-4819-141-11-200412070-00008

3 Greer SM, Goldstein AN, et al. The impact of sleep deprivation on food desire in the human brain. *Nature Communications.* 2013 Aug;4(2259). doi.org/10.1038/ncomms3259

4 Greer. The impact of sleep deprivation on food desire in the human brain.

5 Kallestad H, Hansen B, et al. Impact of sleep disturbance on patients in treatment for mental disorders. *BMC Psychiatry.* 2012 Oct;12(179). doi.org/10.1186/1471-244X-12-179

6 Scott AJ, Webb TL, et al. Does improving sleep lead to better mental health? A protocol for a meta-analytic review of randomised controlled trials. *BMJ Open.* 2017 Sep;7(9). doi.org/10.1136/bmjopen-2017-016873

7 Spiegel. Brief communication.

8 Dye L, Blundell JE. Menstrual cycle and appetite control: implications for weight regulation. *Human Reproduction.* 1997 Jun;12(6):1142–51. doi.org/10.1093/humrep/12.6.1142

Chapter 9

1 Warneken F, Tomasello M. Altruistic Helping in Human Infants and Young Chimpanzees. *Science.* 2006 Mar;311(5765):1301–3. doi.org/10.1126/science.1121448

Chapter 10

1 Calitri R, Pothos EM, et al. Cognitive Biases to Healthy and Unhealthy Food Words Predict Change in BMI. *Obesity.* 2010 Dec;18(12):2282–7. doi.org/10.1038/oby.2010.78

2   Dombrowski. Behavioural Interventions for Obese Adults with Additional Risk Factors for Morbidity.

3   Johns Hopkins University Bloomberg School of Public Health. Home cooking a main ingredient in healthier diet, study shows. *ScienceDaily.* 2014 Nov. sciencedaily.com/releases/2014/11/141117084711.htm

Chapter 11

1   Buettner D. *The Blue Zones.* Washington: National Geographic Society, 2010

2   Aune D, Keum N, et al. Whole grain consumption and risk of cardiovascular disease, cancer, and all cause and cause specific mortality: systematic review and dose-response meta-analysis of prospective studies. *BMJ.* 2016 Jun;353:i2716. doi.org/10.1136/bmj.i2716

3   Deng F. The gut microbiome of healthy long-living people.

PART 3
Chapter 13

1   Skouteris H, McCabe M, et al. Parent–child interactions and obesity prevention: a systematic review of the literature. *Early Child Development and Care.* 2012 Feb;182(2):153–74. doi.org/10.1080/03004430.2010.548606

2   Center for Substance Abuse Treatment. *Tip 57: Trauma-Informed Care in Behavioral Health Services.* Rockville: Substance Abuse and Mental Health Services Administration, 2014. ncbi.nlm.nih.gov/books/NBK207191/box/part1_ch3.box16

3   Mason SM, Flint AJ, et al. Posttraumatic Stress Disorder Symptoms and Food Addiction in Women by Timing and Type of Trauma Exposure. *JAMA Psychiatry.* 2014 Sep;71(11):1271–8. doi.org/10.1001/jamapsychiatry.2014.1208

4   Ibid.

5   Gomez F, Kilpela LS, et al. Sexual trauma uniquely associated with eating disorders: A replication study. *Psychological Trauma: Theory, Research, Practice, and Policy.* 2021;13(2):202–5. doi.org/10.1037/tra0000586

6   Holmes SC, Johnson NL, et al. Understanding the relationship between interpersonal trauma and disordered eating: An extension of the model of psychological adaptation. *Psychological Trauma: Theory, Research, Practice, and Policy.* 2019;14(7):1175–83. doi.org/10.1037/tra0000533

Chapter 14

1   Oxford English Dictionary. *Oxford University Press.* public.oed.com

2   Alda A, Vedantam S. Hidden Brain: Alan Alda Wants Us To Have Better Conversations. *NPR.* 2018 Jan. npr.org/transcripts/577433687

3   UNC Gillings School of Global Public Health. Survey finds disordered eating behaviors among three out of four American women (Fall, 2008). *Carolina Public Health Magazine.* 2008 Sep. sph.unc.edu/cphm/carolina-public-health-magazine-accelerate-fall-2008/survey-finds-disordered-eating-behaviors-among-three-out-of-four-american-women-fall-2008

4   American Academy of Facial Plastic and Reconstructive Surgery, Inc. AAFPRS announces annual survey results: demand for facial plastic surgery skyrockets as pandemic drags on (press release). 2022 Feb. aafprs.org/Media/Press_Releases/2021%20Survey%20Results.aspx

5   Sharp G. Flawed perceptions. *InPsych*. 2018 Jun;40(3):16–21. psychology.org. au/for-members/publications/inpsych/2018/june-issue-3/flawed-perceptions

Chapter 16

1   UNC Gillings School of Global Public Health. Survey finds disordered eating behaviors among three out of four American women (Fall, 2008).
2   Lowes J, Tiggemann M. Body dissatisfaction, dieting awareness and the impact of parental influence in young children. *British Journal of Health Psychology*, 2003 May;8(2),135–47. doi.org/10.1348/135910703321649123
3   Solmi F, Sharpe H, et al. Changes in the Prevalence and Correlates of Weight-Control Behaviors and Weight Perception in Adolescents in the UK, 1986-2015. *JAMA Pediatrics*. 2021 Mar;175(3):267–75. doi.org/10.1001/jamapediatrics.2020.4746
4   Stice E, Gau JM, et al. Risk factors that predict future onset of each *DSM-5* eating disorder: Predictive specificity in high-risk adolescent females. *Journal of Abnormal Psychology*. 2017 Jan;126(1):38–51. doi.org/10.1037/abn0000219 & Litmanen J, Fröjd S, et al. Are eating disorders and their symptoms increasing in prevalence among adolescent population? *Nordic Journal of Psychiatry*. 2017 Jan;71(1):61–6. doi.org/10.1080/08039488.2016.1224272
5   Solmi. Changes in the Prevalence and Correlates of Weight-Control Behaviors and Weight Perception in Adolescents in the UK, 1986-2015.
6   Ibid.
7   Ibid.
8   Ibid.
9   Butterfly. *The Butterfly Foundation*. butterfly.org.au
10 Wansink B, Latimer LA, et al. 'Don't eat so much': how parent comments relate to female weight satisfaction. *Eating and Weight Disorders – Studies on Anorexia, Bulimia and Obesity*. 2017 Sep;22(3):475–81. doi.org/10.1007/s40519-016-0292-6
11 Pesch MH, Miller AL, et al. Mothers of Obese Children Use More Direct Imperatives to Restrict Eating. *Journal of Nutrition Education and Behavior*. 2018 Apr;50(4):403–7. doi.org/10.1016/j.jneb.2017.10.010
12 Wansink. 'Don't eat so much'.
13 Ibid.
14 Eisenberg ME, Berge JM, et al. Associations between hurtful weight-related comments by family and significant other and the development of disordered eating behaviors in young adults. *Journal of Behavioral Medicine*. 2012 Oct;35(5):500–8. doi.org/10.1007/s10865-011-9378-9
15 Neumark-Sztainer. Obesity, disordered eating, and eating disorders in a longitudinal study of adolescents.
16 Spence AC, Campbell KJ, et al. Early Childhood Vegetable, Fruit, and Discretionary Food Intakes Do Not Meet Dietary Guidelines, but Do Show Socioeconomic Differences and Tracking over Time. *Journal of the Academy of Nutrition and Dietetics*. 2018 Sep;118(9):1634–43. doi.org/10.1016/j.jand.2017.12.009

Index

5:2 diet 100
12-week body challenges 17, 203,
    210, 237
1200 calorie diet 28, 32, 152

A

abstinence groups 130
acceptance 31, 45, 69, 103, 105–7,
    110, 153, 166, 168–9, 179–82, 184,
    235, 246, 254–5, 260–2
alcohol 47, 49–50, 53, 82–3, 97, 105,
    119–20, 130, 137, 159, 186
alkaline water 220
all-or-nothing approach 14, 36, 43,
    62, 156–7, 188, 215, 282
American diet industry 27
anorexia 247
anxiety 56–7, 61, 65, 85, 105, 115,
    129, 173, 181, 184, 192, 227
app, Back to Basics 37, 150, 279
appetite 46, 80, 85, 129, 144–6, 148,
    150–3, 157–8, 161, 197, 206, 227,
    274–5, 277–8, 284
    see also hunger
Atkins diet 33, 221, 231

B

Back to Basics app 37, 150, 279
basic needs 73–4, 76–83, 88, 96–7,
    112, 122, 170, 202
beauty standards 53, 58
before-and-after photos 32, 34, 58,
    67, 203–4, 210
binge eating 11–12, 43, 45, 67, 79,
    103, 125, 127, 130–1, 135, 136–9,
    146, 153, 157, 169, 230, 247, 276
biomarkers 56
blame *see* self-blame
blood pressure 54, 56, 63, 118
blood sugar levels 54
blood tests 63–4, 115, 155, 207
Blue Zones 213
body
    body acceptance 69

body fat *see* fat, body
body goals *see* goals
body hatred 18, 30–1, 45, 58–60,
    247, 251, 256–7, 260–1, 263,
    265, 273, 276, 281
body image 10–11, 18, 23, 47, 65,
    162, 229, 231, 233, 240, 252,
    254–8, 264, 268–70, 272–3,
    277, 282
body love 53, 102–3, 109, 163, 166,
    247, 254–5, 261
body positive movement 53
body shame 233, 271, 282–3
body, relationship with 10, 14, 45,
    103, 107, 129, 269, 274
Body Mass Index (BMI) 10, 16, 25,
    52–5, 57, 60, 210, 272–3, 276
boredom 137, 148, 205, 277, 283
boundaries 173, 181–4, 232–5
bowels 104, 121, 160
    bowel movements 40, 64–5, 158,
    160
brains 26–9, 34–6, 45, 48, 57, 69, 72,
    85, 96–7, 116, 118, 121, 130, 132,
    134, 136, 144–5, 153, 156, 158,
    163, 166, 168, 175, 180, 209, 243,
    246, 257, 262, 268, 284
bread 35, 131–4, 138, 140, 146, 151,
    170
breakfast 103, 133, 135, 146, 152,
    250
burnout 13–4, 113–15, 135, 176,
    178, 186, 205
    diet burnout 10, 14, 42, 44–5, 47,
    114, 127, 137, 145

C

calcium 97, 140, 152
calories 12, 15, 28, 33, 35, 45, 68–9,
    87, 89, 96, 105–6, 123, 126,
    131–2, 138–9, 145–6, 150–3,
    155–5, 167, 190–1, 193–6, 204,
    207, 211, 215, 286
calorie deficit 24

overeating 29, 45, 103, 129, 134–5, 137, 139, 156, 169, 207, 275
perfect eating 14, 106, 134, 198–9
relationship with food 9–12, 14–19, 21, 25, 27, 36, 61, 100, 122–41, 145, 155–6, 193, 208, 212, 226–8, 231, 233, 235, 237, 239–40, 243, 271–4, 283–4, 286–7, 289
satisfying foods 131–5, 155–6
skipping meals 34, 48, 79, 133, 221
snake-meals 132–3, 135
structured eating 44
superfoods 35, 213
undereating 58, 76, 79, 123, 125, 135, 156, 159, 203, 237, 256
updating your food language 274–7
weighing 10, 58, 128, 148, 231
forgiveness 18, 49–50, 109–10, 166, 232, 261–3
fridge, reorganising 200
fruit 35, 38, 64, 77, 82, 89, 97–8, 127, 132–3, 146, 200, 213–15, 221, 285
fattening myth 214
fullness 39, 68, 85–6, 97, 104, 129, 131, 134, 141–3, 147–50, 157, 162, 196, 277–8, 284–5

G
gastric sleeves 31
ghrelin 155–6, 158, 162
glucose 130
gluten 33, 35, 40, 127, 159, 219–20
glycogen 130
goals 18, 47, 49, 56, 64–6, 74–5, 91, 102, 106, 154, 160, 168, 178, 263, 280
body goals 66, 106, 251, 261
fitness goal 64, 87, 99, 106, 204, 207
goal weight 12, 14–5, 37, 45, 47, 57–9, 61, 100, 191
health goals 64–6, 69, 109, 191, 263
setting gentle goals 102–3
weight-loss goals 37, 60–2, 191, 260, 286

guilt 9, 12, 18, 30, 34–5, 37, 44, 48–51, 68, 79, 97, 104, 109, 115, 123, 127–9, 135, 138–40, 154–7, 167, 176–7, 192–3, 206, 208, 210–12, 214–15, 225, 228, 236–7, 247, 249, 256, 278
reframing 51
guts 121, 144, 147, 158, 215, 219, 250
gut health 89, 203, 213–14
gut microbiota 214

H
habits 47, 69, 71, 77, 86, 88, 135, 146, 158, 160, 166, 174–5, 178, 188–200, 209, 218–9, 234–6, 266, 282, 284, 287
building on existing habits 101–3
core habits 83–8, 97, 142, 164, 189, 202, 217
eating habits 25, 230, 239, 278
enrichment habits 88–92, 98, 202–15
habit gaps 76–8, 80–81, 83–4, 88, 90, 92, 95–6, 108, 145
healthy 13, 16–17, 19, 28, 37, 40, 46, 49, 60–1, 67, 69, 74–93, 95–104, 107–8, 118, 142, 162, 189–91, 195, 204–5, 207, 209–10, 216–17, 219, 228, 238, 268, 271, 284, 286
hierarchy of healthy habits 50, 69, 74–93, 95–6, 108, 112, 122, 136, 142, 164, 170, 189, 194, 204, 207, 212, 216–17, 269
ideal habits 92–3, 216–21
testing new habits 95–101
unhealthy 61, 99, 139, 230
hair loss 53, 79
happiness 23–4, 31, 62, 64–5, 68, 106, 114, 116, 124, 156, 168, 173, 182, 210, 246, 255, 261, 263–4, 269, 286
see also unhappiness
headaches 56, 64, 120, 147
health 11–19, 32–4, 37–40, 42, 44–8, 50–8, 60, 71, 74–80, 82–3, 86, 88–9, 91–5, 99, 104–9, 112, 114–15, 117–18, 129, 135, 140,